W9-BGI-311

Hold Me Tight

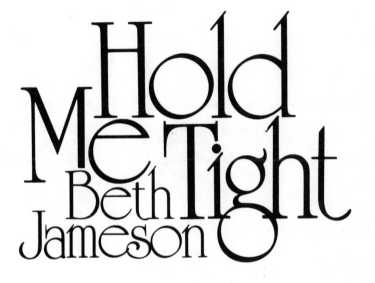

Hold Me Tight

Beth Jameson

Fleming H. Revell Company
Old Tappan, New Jersey

Library of Congress Cataloging in Publication Data

Jameson, Beth.
  Hold me tight.

  1. Leukemia in children—Patients—Colorado—
Biography.   2. Jameson, Kim.   3. Christian biog-
raphy—Colorado.   I. Title.
RJ416.L4J35   248.4   80-36821
ISBN 0-8007-1129-7

Contents

Preface

"To bury a child is to see a part of yourself—your eye color, your dimple, your sense of humor—being placed in the ground. It is life's harshest empathetic experience and must therefore be the hardest one with which to deal. In reality, when children die, not only are we mourning them, we are also mourning that bit of our own immortality that they carried" (Harriet Shiff).

The day I knelt in the dirt at the open grave of my daughter, in the misty phantoms of pained reality, was the day I knew those serene days of trusting in an unchallenged faith were over. "To die must be an awfully big adventure," said Peter Pan, but accepting the challenge to continue after the death of one's child is an even greater one. For, when my child was buried, a part of me was also placed into the ground. Death is the ultimate loss. The death of one's child is the ultimate tragedy. I am stunned by thoughts of what could have been and will never be.

This book was wrought through irreconcilable grief. In my desperate search to unscramble feelings, thoughts, and questions, writing became a tool to cope with death's stark intrusion. It began as a means of soul washing, a pouring out of feelings when there were no longer ears that would listen. Healthy grief work was mistakenly postponed when the diagnosis of leukemia struck again. Our home added my mother-in-law and subtracted my child with the same destructive denominator: leukemia. In the awesome process of managing this additional tragedy, my intolerable sense of loss could not find expression. Grief was more than just a rip in the fabric of my life. It became a gaping hole very loosely patched. The reweaving did not begin for a long time. Courage for another was still needed. So the frustrations of being unable to work through my grief became a lonesome torture. I was together on the outside, but my inner self remained in shambles. When I did not respond to the timetable of acceptable grief set by others, support was withdrawn. I cherish the relationships of those who patiently stood by me until the metamorphosis was complete.

As the torn strands of emotional calamity are slowly being rewoven, I have finally achieved a healthy sense of gratitude for this searing encounter with an all-knowing, all-powerful, ever-present God. The power of a rechallenged faith has taken my sorrow and changed it into a depth of character and achievement that would never have been realized otherwise. Only in grief can the human spirit plumb the depths of its existence, comprehend life's meaning, and emerge scarred but triumphant. The depth of grief I have reached has served as a rising point to a higher, more meaningful, level of living. It has been worth all enduring. The pain and pleasure of knowing Him has left me with a solid faith in a trustworthy God. My life is now a doxology. How I underestimated my ability to survive!

I will be eternally grateful for the many friends who shared each agonizing stage of Kim's illness with us—especially for the caring love of the congregations of the First Baptist Church of New Orleans, Louisiana, and the Willowmeadows Baptist Church of Houston, Texas. They kept our spirits planted in a realistic perspective. Their supportive prayers carried us through the valley, when we were stopped in our tracks.

To Dr. Taru Hays, Mary Jo Clapp, and the oncology staff of Children's Hospital, Denver, Colorado, our deepest gratitude for being motivated by a love for Kim to go far beyond scientific expectations to halt the destructive force of leukemia. Nothing was spared until the cupboard of medical science was bare and death unleashed its final blow. Clinical roles were dropped and withdrawn with the needles of dashed hopes as unabashed love and grief flowed between just good friends.

A special thank-you to my friend and mentor Dr. Victor Oliver, who recognized with incisive insight the need for such a book to be published when this manuscript from an unknown, unpublished manuscript landed, unsolicited, on his desk. Only through his encouragement, patience, and unrelenting support did these pages ever come to life. Because of him, writing is a brand-new discovery, "God's extra touch," in my life, and a brand-new adventure in following Him.

And, finally, my love and gratitude to the two persons who lived the dying with me every day: my husband, Jim, and our son, Jame. Though we did not have each other for comfort, we shared the true meaning of infinite loneliness and emotional isolation that only the death of a child can bring to a parent and sibling. Grief is a nonsharing emotion. We each carry it alone and in our own way. And thus it will ever be.

Foreword

This book is a very private look at a real family in great crises, a family with an incredible commitment to God. But it's much more!

This is a book that if we allow it:

> Immeasurably escalates our growing experience
>
> Provides us with courage to embrace each day with joy
>
> Prepares us, when life is both ecstatically lovely and hideously painful, to endure victoriously
>
> And finally presents us with enough viable examples that we are able to trust and see, firsthand, the sovereignty of God.

We need nothing more from any book!

JOYCE LANDORF

Hold Me Tight

1

Homestretch to Heaven

"I'M AFRAID IT'S LEUKEMIA." With these words, Dr. Charles August, director of the Department of Hematology at Children's Hospital, pulls the pin on the grenade of our lives.

"Oh, my God, no!" I grasp Dr. August's arm as he sits on the edge of a desk. "Please, please, you've *got* to be mistaken! Kim's never been sick a day in her life! It just can't be. No, no, no! Jim!" I collapse in my husband's arms like a marionette whose strings have been cut. I hear the screeching, grinding agony of my world crashing around me. Fear drops over us like a heavy wet blanket. My throat becomes clogged with frozen screams.

My God, we just walked into this conference room five minutes ago. And I popped off a flippant remark, on seeing so many doctors, "Well, it must be pretty important, Jim. The whole shootin' match is here!" Five minutes, that's all it took: five minutes, and four words.

There seems no way for our prayers to escape this conference room. The awful reality of what they are telling us begins to sink in. Dear God, I don't even know what they're talking about! *Leukemia.* Help me to focus on what they're saying.

"We have agreed," Dr. August is saying, "on the diagnosis of acute lymphocytic leukemia [ALL]. This type of leukemia is a childhood disease of the blood-forming organs: the bone marrow, lymph nodes, and spleen. Let me explain as simply as possible what it is and how it will affect Kim. Her blood-forming tissues are manufacturing false white cells—leukemic cells—that are disrupting the normal production of red blood cells, which prevent anemia; white blood cells, which fight infection; and production of platelets, which control blood clotting and prevent hemorrhages. And she is suffering accordingly. The bone-marrow aspiration we did yesterday provided the conclusive evidence. There is no known way to prevent leukemia, nor can we speak in terms of a cure—only in terms of control, through a combined use of antileukemic drugs and radiation therapy."

His words form a tight, hard ball in my mind, which begins to bounce out of control, down a dark, narrow corridor to the depths of my soul. It picks up speed as it pounds against doors that keep slamming shut—doors that spell hope, life, laughter, a future. God help us.

I think of Kim, down the hall in room 374. That bright, fun-loving, soon-to-be teenager, with long, thick pigtails hanging over her pillow. She is watching TV, waiting for us to come back, apprehensive because the doctors wanted to talk to Jim and me alone. Oh, God, she's somehow got to be told why her legs and back are hurting. How?

My soul is drowning in tears. I don't even recognize the sounds of my own anguish. Jim drops his glasses on the floor and takes me in his arms, with unspeakable sadness.

God, You're surely making a monstrous mistake! What could Your purpose possibly be? Why, God—*why?*

It is very strange suddenly to realize that, from a certain moment on, one's life will never be the same. One's dreams cease, and only existence becomes important. I feel a gentle touch on my shoulder.

"Mrs. Jameson, let me talk to Kim for you. She's old enough to know the truth, and she's too bright to be fooled. It will be easier if we are honest right from the start." I raise my pounding head.

Through blurred vision, I see, for the first time, hematologist Dr. Taru Hays. Her compelling East India accent charms each word she speaks. "As well as being her doctor, I'll be her friend. I want to be yours, too."

I feel drawn to Dr. Hays, and I know Kim will, too. For the next three years she is to be our link between life and death. Thank You for this, God.

"Yes, please, Dr. Hays. She's probably wondering what's taking us so long. I just can't face her yet."

As the doctors and nurses leave, I feel as if Jim and I are stranded on a ruined battlefield. Remnants of a happy life and dreams of a bright future lie scattered and broken around us, in jagged pieces of uncertainty.

Fact and truth overtake my refusal to believe. Grief and helpless fear become uninvited residents in my soul. They are to be tenants, coming and going at will. But no matter how long their absence, I know they will return. The lease is long-term and binding.

Jim breaks the silence. "Beth, we've got to go to Kim. And not like this. We can't help her if we look defeated."

Strength, from what I will learn is a "faith reserve," pulls me together. But I feel like a cardboard cutout, from a carefully planned pattern of creation, walking outside the realm of order. My movements are purely mechanical. To be told one minute my child has a fatal disease and the next minute blow my nose, put on lipstick and a smile, and walk calmly to her room—how can I? How can I face her? How can I look into her eyes? What can I say and remain emotionally in control, when my heart is pounding like a relentless pneumatic drill, boring down to the depths of my soul?

Yet here I go, groping the slick, yellow-plastered walls of that hall, as if I were blind. What I really feel like doing is screaming my head off. But I don't. Instead, I take a deep breath. We walk calmly into her room.

Dr. Hays is still there. Kim's face reflects fear as she reaches for my hand. The whole world has changed since I last saw her.

"Mom, Dr. Hays says I have something called lu-lu-ke-mia." She stumbles over the unfamiliar word.

"I know, darling, but don't be afraid. Just do everything Dr. Hays says, and you'll make it just fine." I don't know how, I only know she must! She begins to cry as I hold her and comfort her. Jim's arms settle around both of us.

We listen together as Dr. Hays begins to explain the method of treatment and drugs Kim will immediately be starting. She also has to tell us that Kim might experience unpleasant side effects from the drugs, including hair loss. *Hair loss!* Now, really, God, this is hardly fair!

Kim looks horrified, an expression I have never before seen on her face. She grabs each pigtail, locking her slim fingers around them. *"No!* Who ever heard of a bald-headed teenager? Oh, mother. I'll never have any more friends. I just want to go ahead and die right now!"

That evening Jim and I drive the unfamiliar route to our home, in Littleton, from Children's Hospital, in downtown Denver. We moved here only six days ago, from Louisiana. Jim's hands clutch the wheel, and I sit beside him as though I had just been told to "freeze" in a childhood game. My fingers curl tightly around two new booklets in my lap: *Childhood Leukemia,* a pamphlet for parents, and *Oncology Information for Parents.* I don't even know what *oncology* means.

The big Mayflower moving van is just pulling away from the curb, the movers having done as much as they can with no one home. Jim fumbles for the key to the front door. We step from a daze into a maze: moving boxes piled everywhere, no place to relax. No familiar walls comfort us. No familiar faces greet us.

Jim plugs in the refrigerator. It struggles to respond, as though it knows it's out of place there in the middle of the kitchen floor.

Finally it settles into a lovely, familiar hum. I never appreciated that hum so much before. It sounds like the reassuring voice of an old friend, in this strange, echoing house.

Our sixteen-year-old son, Jame, comes in the front door, breathless from the drastic change in altitude and from trying out for the football team at his new school, Arapahoe High.

"Hey, where's Kim?"

And so began the drama that, in three years, would change our lives and reach a shattering, climactic revelation with the last page in Kim's diary, written Thanksgiving Day, 1975:

> **November 27** I woke up at 2:30 and began thinkin'. No one can hurt this bad and be the least bit well. I'm so confused. Help me, God! I believe I'm on the homestretch to heaven.

2

Beginning a Long Road

THE DAY HAD COME when, suddenly, what always happens to someone else happened to us. On August 23, 1973, we were in a strange city we knew nothing about, on a street we had to look for on a map, miles away from our friends and family. Only six days had led us to this destination; it was a trip that began with a search through the Yellow Pages, under "Physicians–Hospitals," because Kim was not feeling well, en route to Denver. That was my first indication something might be wrong. August 4 was Kim's first indication.

> **August 4**   Karen Browning and I got up at 5:30 to go bike riding. It was fun, but my leg and side are still bothering me. I don't know what's the matter. All I know is that they hurt! We went to Aunt Sister's house and rested. She made us biscuits and syrup, and that tasted so good. I'm just so tired. Last night I woke up with my leg and side hurting me so much I could hardly walk. It hurts so badly!

Kim and Jame were staying with their grandmother in Plainview, Texas. Jim and I had been in Denver, buying a house, and were now back in Louisiana, working with the movers and packing. On August 15 we went to pick up the children. Kim seemed especially glad to see me. She had tears in her eyes, when we hugged each other.

"Mother, I haven't been feeling good at all. I'm so glad you're here!"

We walked into our new house, in Littleton, August 19. Before Jame and Kim finished their inspection, a big Mayflower moving van groaned its way around the corner and stopped in front.

By midafternoon I suspected Kim was running a fever. I asked the movers to please set up her bed as soon as possible. A quiet panic set in. I didn't even know where a drugstore was, much less a doctor! Aspirin didn't seem to help. We spent a restless, exhausting night.

The next morning, with the aid of a map and a telephone directory, I located the nearest doctor's office. Kim looked awful.

"C'mon, babe," I told her. "Let's go find some help." I helped her to the car, and she lay on the backseat. With the phone book beside me, we started out. After making two stops, I realized all the doctors were swamped with before-school examinations.

Finally, at the Littleton Clinic, the receptionist agreed to squeeze Kim in after the doctors were finished for the day. I gathered Kim up like a limp dishrag.

The afternoon passed quickly. It was soon time to go back to the clinic. Kim was so weak. Was it the heat, or was her temperature getting higher?

After the doctor examined her, he called me into his office. He was suspicious of some of the test results.

Kim wrote in her diary that night:

> **August 19**   Mom took me to a doctor to see about my leg and side. They took blood tests and X rays, and the doctor said I'm going to have to go to the Children's Hospital. I'm scared half to death!

August 21—it was so cool and peaceful early in the morning. God, if I could just stay half awake for a little while longer. But the curtain of a new day was quickly parting, again revealing the pressures of the previous day and bringing to light the tasks of this day. I was not even up, and already I felt weighted. I had to thank You first, God—and fast! Then I asked for Your help in handling whatever situation awaited us in the day's passing.

The telephone installer was supposed to come at 9:00, so Jim took Kim to the hospital. Kim carried her purse, but not an overnight bag. We didn't consider the possibility of her having to stay. She was quiet and noticeably worried as she followed Jim out the front door. I reached out to hold her warm face close to mine and give her a smooch.

"Don't worry, babe, I'll come the minute the phone man is through."

Jame gulped breakfast down in a hurry. He had a busy, important day ahead of him, too, getting started in another new school—the fifth in only four years. It was also his first year in high school.

He stopped at the front door. "Don't worry, mom. Dad'll probably have Kim back home before you get there."

Little did I know, two hours later, as I drove toward the distant, tall buildings of downtown Denver, that this was to be only the first of many trips. I felt so alone. Dear God, I prayed, help me.

We did not bring Kim home that evening, nor for another week—a week that shattered our life-style and broke our hearts.

Thank You, Lord, for a sense of humor. I wore it threadbare, keeping Kim from being afraid during her first stay in a hospital: making jokes with the doctors and nurses; bringing Kim whimsical flower arrangements; drawing ladybugs and daisies, with magic markers, on her arms, where the lab technician would draw blood; writing poems and notes, to send to the dietician, on the food tray. Together, our inventive wheels turned very well!

One day Kim made a sign on a sheet of paper and taped it to the head of her bed. It read: PLEASE DO NOT FEED THE PATIENTS. THEY'RE SICK ENOUGH AS IT IS!

> **August 22**   Woke up at 7:00 and ate breakfast. It's kind of fun to mark the menus, but the food is just fair. Dad came about 8:30, on his way to work. Mom called me on the phone, and then she came about noon. Today they took some more blood tests—ugh! But the worst thing was a bone-marrow test. The doctors explained to me what it was before they did it, but they could never explain how much it was going to hurt! It hurt me more than anything in my whole life. They brought me back to my room in a wheelchair. I was so glad to see mom waitin' by my bed. Hope I sleep better tonight. They take my temperature too much.

Kim underwent test after test, all their procedures and names so foreign from anything we had ever heard of before. She had always been the picture of health, our cheerleader! I shifted into a gear I didn't know I had, in order to handle the mounting pressures of each day.

Every evening the mailbox was full of notes from servicemen whose appointments I missed by needing to be at the hospital longer than I planned.

This strange roller coaster of trials kept picking up speed and problems. For, in the next few weeks, our basement flooded, with all these stacked boxes everywhere; the washing machine motor burned out; the furnace went out on the day the temperature dropped to four degrees and Jim was out of town; the picture tube went out on the TV; a plumbing leak developed in the upstairs bathroom, ruining the flooring and damaging the living-room ceiling; a gust of wind slammed the back storm door against the house and broke the glass; the vinyl dashboard on my car cracked in four places during a long, cold night; I broke a filling on a tooth and turned over a gallon of white paint on the kitchen floor. And for the first time in eighteen years, we got a notice from the Internal Revenue Service that they wanted to audit our income taxes for the last four years.

A long-distance call came from a friend in Houston, "Hey, how do y'all like Denver?"

3

Home Again

"YOU CAN GO HOME TODAY, Kim." At last! A chance of getting back to normal, being a family again, living again, away from the reminders of never again being the same! My ability to rebel against an unsolvable reality that hurt begins to emerge once more.

One is supposed to feel relief, getting out of a hospital—right? The body is healing, on the road back to health. Whatever caused the interruption that turned person into patient is left behind. The hospital, the doctors, the nurses—they eradicated the problem. It is no more.

That's the way it's *supposed* to be. But it seems as if nothing is the way it's supposed to be anymore. We didn't leave something behind at the hospital. We're bringing something home with us: Something that doesn't belong, something we didn't know existed this time last week! How can normal living patterns resume, when something so abnormal has infiltrated those patterns?

Each of us will have to adjust to a radically altered situation of normalcy. *How*, God? It surely will cause unavoidable changes in attitudes and behavior in each of us, just in the management of daily living. *Why*, God?

And if God cares so wonderfully for flowers that are here today and gone tomorrow, won't he surely care for you, O

27

men of little faith? . . . So don't be anxious about tomorrow. God will take care of your tomorrow too. Live one
day at a time.

Matthew 6:30, 34

Live one day at a time. . . . Live one day at a time. . . . Those six
words form a chain of constant restraint, keeping my faith intact
and my mind from leaping impulsively ahead into tomorrow's
abyss of hopelessness. Just repeating those words over and over
helps me to remember that God is still in control. Hearing them,
reading them, brings a serenity over my being and quiets my
soul, when I so quickly become engulfed in the "what in the
world are we going to do" of tomorrow. They become my verbal
tranquilizer.

It's a quiet drive home, with Kim sitting beside me in the car,
our separate thoughts blocking out the noise of city traffic. Soon
Kim begins to talk about what needs to be done before school
starts—about clothes, classes, teachers, as if this past week were
just a horrible nightmare, now over. God, if it only were!

Jim is already home, having driven his car ahead of us. Jame
should be home soon. The garage is too cluttered to put the car
in, so we stop in the driveway.

"Mom, I wish we were back in Louisiana."

The front door closes behind us. We are met with self-pity,
loneliness, helplessness, and despondency—all enemies that are
part of the battle we will learn to fight as part of each day's routine. Shock sets in. There is no pill, no drug, *nothing* to relieve our
wounded spirits. ". . . my sadness and troubles were weighed . . .
they are heavier than the sand of a thousand seashores. . ." (Job
6:2, 3).

God, I feel as if I'm losing my sense of survival! I feel like a
coach who has to be a competitor, too, in order for there to be a
contest at all. Kim is running a race, and I'm her teammate. I
don't have the strength, do I? Does she? It's really like running a

race against time and circumstance, not knowing if the finish line will be around the corner of tomorrow or a year of tomorrows. One of us won't finish at all.

I must pace myself, take a deep breath, plan my strategy, plot the game plan. Surely this first lap of shock will be the hardest. It's *got* to slack up. I must give Kim the incentive to keep running, at whatever pace, at whatever cost. She must develop the will to run without the flag of victory in sight. Is that possible?

C'mon, baby! I'm right beside you. We're a team now. Run! Reach out for that relay stick of hope, when it comes back around. Grab it! Hang on! *Go!* . . . "Forgetting the past and looking forward to what lies ahead, I strain to reach the end of the race and receive the prize for which God is calling . . ." (Philippians 3:13, 14).

> **August 27** Worked on my room as much as I could. It was a real hot day, and I didn't feel like doing much. What made the day nice was getting some flowers from the Lands, in New Orleans, and a real cute purse from Mrs. Adkins. I'm so homesick for our friends. Why did all this have to happen? I can't think of anything so bad that I've done. And we're all Christians, too. Talked to mom a long time. I asked her to let me see what the encyclopedia said on leukemia. I want to know everything about what I've got. She brought me the stuff to read, but told me not to worry, because the information was out of date. But it says I could *die* from this! How can I keep from worrying?

There's a knock at the back door. "Hello, I'm Helen Wendorff, your neighbor across the street. I haven't been able to catch you at home, and one of the movers told me you were at the hospital, with your daughter. Is there anything I can do to help? What's the matter? Nothing serious, I hope."

Throughout the struggle, Helen Wendorff will become the caring, compassionate, do-anything-for-you neighbor we need.

"Well, yes. Our daughter has leukemia." There! I said it! I popped the cork on our pressurized bottle of secrecy! It exploded without restraint, spewing bitterness and hidden guilt. I didn't care. Go ahead, world, spread the vicious news! My child has leukemia. *My child has leukemia.* My . . . child . . . has . . . leukemia. And I . . . can't . . . help it.

I had said "that word" aloud to a stranger. My voice was barely audible, yet the sound of that word carried a thunderous shout. I feel an enormous wave of relief, but also a biting repulsion and guilt one would associate with leprosy, as if our whole family should be quarantined, isolated from the community.

An electric expression flashes across my neighbor's face, as she manages to speak. "Oh, I'm so sorry! Let me give you my phone number, and, if you need anything, be sure to call me."

She quickly leaves, as if she were interfering. She was not prepared for such a blunt answer. She expected a flu-recover, not a cancer-death, answer. It is my first encounter with the average person's inability to accept and understand another person's involvement in a life-death situation.

The homecoming is not easy. Kim's condition is very uncertain. The goal of remission is yet to be reached. Feelings of hostility have to be dealt with. Patience and understanding have to be exercised beyond their straining points, in order to meet the responsibilities of everyday life. No, the coming home is not easy.

Jim hands me a little blue card he was given before leaving the hospital. It indicates Kim will be an outpatient in the oncology clinic at Children's, as long as she successfully responds to the treatments. I slip it into a plastic division of my billfold, next to a never-used in-case-of-emergency card. Being an outpatient means that numerous, regular trips to the hospital will become a big part of our routine of living. It also means that having Kim home as much as possible will give us a better chance to become a normal, happy family again. To me, it is also a chance to escape

from the heart-wrenching world of the terminally sick and suffering within the walls of the hospital—a world that all too soon
will become our world.

The time we spend going back and forth to the hospital is not
wasted. They are precious, private times—a sharing of each
others' thoughts, anxieties, and pain. We even have fun experi-
menting with new routes, shortcuts, getting lost and finding our
way again. We become so familiar with so many different ways
to get to the hospital that we joke about Orleans, our car, being
able to get us there on her own. All one has to do is push the
button on the dash, marked CHILDREN'S HOSPITAL!

But no matter how jovial we are on the way, how successfully
our spirits are launched, a heavy cloud of fear descends over us
as I drive into the parking lot in front of the hospital. The tail
ends of chattering sentences trail off into meaningless silence.
Each time we press down on those polished steel levers opening
the big glass doors at the entrance and step on that red carpet,
my heart sinks. *This* is reality: it cannot be erased. Neither can
our presence. The choice is not ours to make.

We turn to the right and walk up the pink-veined-marble
steps, to the second floor. Through the main lobby, around the
curve of the business-office window, a stop at the water fountain,
then we proceed down the highly polished vinyl-tile floor of a
very long hall. Near the end, across from the gray steel doors of
the elevator, is a sign on the left wall: ONCOLOGY CLINIC. Underneath is a directional arrow, pointing straight ahead. Although
attractive paintings are hung above the tiled wainscoting and
bustling hospital activity is all around, I will never seem to notice
more than the beige tile squares that disappear under my feet,
during the long walks I take up and down that hall. Each time,
we can always be pretty sure of what to expect in the way of
tests, but are never sure what the results might be, or the treatment to be followed.

The regular routine of clinic procedure becomes to let them

know Kim is there, pick up a slip for the lab, then go back through the clinic waiting room, down the hall to the elevator, and up to the fifth floor, where she will have a blood test made. Then we go back down to the clinic waiting room, to wait. Sitting in that room is like sitting at a big picture window, watching the world struggle by—a time spent in our own private agony. The hollow sounds of children's laughter as they play with toys scattered on the floor seems to mock death. The drone of television does not cover the cries that can so quickly follow a laugh. My brain receives difficult, heartbreaking messages of what my eyes are seeing for the first time in the life-snatching atmosphere of this waiting room. My brain does not want to accept such messages.

Kim and I try to carry on a light conversation, but we hear the muffled cries of a weak, disease-riddled child, nestled in a drained mother's protective arms. My mouth goes dry as we silently watch a gaily painted toy wagon roll by, with a cargo bearing signs of cancer's ruthless attack on an angelic, moon-faced four-year-old. His haunting, blank stare does not reflect the cheerful attitude of the student nurse pulling him around. A wheelchair is pushed by, equipped with an intravenous bottle swinging from a pole. It is occupied by a young girl of about fourteen, encased in the shriveled-up body of a ravaging disease. Only her dark, questioning eyes give the slightest hint of youth.

Kim and I cuddle closer on the blue-vinyl couch. We've somehow got to concentrate on the TV program that's on. Relax, body! By relaxing, it's easier not to see. And if we don't really see, maybe we won't be able to relate. But we can't relax. We never do, really. That waiting room is always a place where time seems to be in suspension and our emotions frozen until Kim's name is called.

Dear God, please spare Kim from the road these precious ones are on. Spare Jim and me from having to walk alongside, so helplessly! There must be another way! There must be a detour! We are so painfully becoming aware of being caught up in this constant parade of horrors all going in the same direction!

"Kim?" The voice belongs to Mary Jo Clapp, coordinator of nursing services in oncology, the registered nurse who will be so skillfully administering the antileukemic drugs to Kim, during the next three years. But she will do so much more than that. She will also administer love, compassion, and understanding that will give us all the will to keep fighting. She will cry and laugh with us. She will listen to us. We always feel her support, regardless of the tenseness of the situation. Mary Jo Clapp—a very special lady—has just become an important part of our lives. She fills in the gap, during the times when, emotionally, I can no longer handle the situation. Kim grows to love and trust her very much. We all do.

It's a relief to leave the waiting room, even though we don't know what experiences might be in store for us back in the clinic. We wait for Dr. Hays in one of the small examining rooms. How familiar we will become with these small rooms. Each one waits to take its turn being the scene of painful, traumatic experiences Kim will have to go through in her fight with leukemia.

Hope is introduced to us in the form of chemotherapy—a method of drug treatment that will keep Kim delicately balanced between life and death. I'm given a typewritten page to study: "Investigational and Conventional Anticancer Drugs and Their Possible Side Effects," for Kim Jameson. My eyes stumble over the progression of letters as my voice struggles to pronounce the strange-sounding names. It's apparent that our vocabulary must change, along with our world. My voice knots with effort, as I slowly proceed down the page:

ADRIAMYCIN—(Doxorubicin or ADR given as an IV shot) Can cause bone marrow depression, mouth sores, nausea and vomiting, hair loss, chemical burn on skin if leakage from the vein occurs, heart changes on electrocardiogram, increased heart rate, red urine.

ALLOPURINOL—(pill, to stop formation of uric acid) Bone marrow depression.

BIS-CHLOROETHYL-NITROSUREA—(BCNU, given as IV shot) Bone marrow depression, decrease in platelets and white blood count, nausea, vomiting, decrease in appetite, chemical burn on skin if leakage occurs.

CYCLOLEUCINE—Loss of appetite, nausea, vomiting, gastrointestinal hemorrhage, anemia, possible aggravation of mild diabetes, bone marrow suppression, diarrhea, infrequent neurologic effects.

CYTOSINE ARABINOSIDE—(Cytosar, Ara-C, given as IV shot or just under the skin. Stops cells from making DNA so they can't divide) May cause liver damage, nausea and vomiting, decrease in appetite, bone marrow depression, stomach cramps, headache, sore throat, decrease in white blood cells, diarrhea.

CYTOXAN—(Cyclophosphamide or CTX, given as pill or IV shot, alkylating agent drug) Bone marrow depression, loss of appetite, nausea, vomiting, hair loss, sores in mouth, diarrhea, decrease in white blood cells and platelets, bleeding from bladder, pain when urinating.

DACTINOMYCIN—Nausea, vomiting, decrease in white blood cells and platelets, hair loss, chemical burn on skin if leakage from vein occurs, increased tanning and redness of skin if used in radiation therapy.

DAUNOMYCIN—(Daunorubricin, Rubidomycin or DNR, IV shot, antibiotic group of drugs, acts by stopping cells from making DNA and RNA so cells cannot grow and divide) Nausea, vomiting, diarrhea, fever, abdominal pain, headache, sores in mouth, hair loss, bone marrow depression, chemical burn on skin if leakage from vein occurs, heart changes on electrocardiogram. Use mouthwash three times daily.

5-Azacytidine—Nausea, vomiting, bone marrow depression, damage to liver.

5-Fluorouracil—(5FU) Decrease in white blood cells and platelets, sores in mouth, diarrhea, ulcers or bleeding in stomach or intestine, bleeding from any site, nausea, vomiting, loss of hair, rashes.

L-Asparaginase—(Asp or L-ASP—given only as shot, IV or IM—in muscle, enzyme group of drugs. Blasts need protein to grow and divide. L-ASP acts by breaking up one of the ingredients blasts need to make protein. Possible sudden allergic reaction, needle must remain in vein approximately half hour after receiving L-ASP) Allergic shock, bone marrow depression, damage to liver and kidneys, nausea, vomiting.

Mercaptopurine—(6MP or Purinethol, either pill or IV shot, an antimetabolite group of drugs—acts by stopping cells from making new DNA so they cannot divide) Sores in mouth, bone marrow depression, nausea and vomiting when given in vein, loss of appetite, diarrhea, liver damage. Use mouthwash three times daily.

Methotrexate—(MTX, given in spinal tap, pill, IV or IM, antimetabolite group of drugs) Sores in mouth, bone marrow depression, hair loss, nausea and vomiting, loss of appetite, rashes, fragile bones, possible liver damage and lung problems. Use mouthwash three times daily.

Prednisone—(PRED, or closely related drug Dexamethasone—Decadron: given as pill only, a hormone like cortisone—only stronger, acts by killing lymphocytes, tapering dosage) Increase in appetite, weight gain, round face, retention of fluids, softening of bones, may provoke latent diabetes or tuberculosis, may cover up symptoms of infection, weakness, high blood sugar, higher blood pressure, mood changes. Decrease salt in diet.

PROCARBAZINE—(Natulan) Nausea, vomiting, decrease in white blood cells and platelets, liver toxicity. Do not give narcotics, sedatives, or Phenathiazine drugs when using this. Dramamine and Pyndoxine may be used to combat nausea.
STREPTOZOTOCIN—Nausea, vomiting, abnormal renal, liver or pancreatic function, bone marrow depression.
VINCRISTINE—(Oncovin or VCR, given only as IV shot, from a group of drugs called vinca alkaloids, comes from the periwinkle plant, acts on dividing cells to stop them from dividing, given once a week at start of induction because not all leukemia cells are dividing at one time) Hair loss, constipation, abdominal cramps, decrease in white blood cells, tingling and numbness in fingers or toes, muscle pain, changes in walking, stumbling, decrease in knee jerks and other reflexes, chemical burn on skin if leakage from vein occurs, weakness. May use laxative.

All of the above drugs will increase susceptibility to infection. Your child will experience few, many, or perhaps none of the above side effects. Your child should drink plenty of liquids while receiving any of the above drugs or radiation therapy, to help clear the system of breakdown products of cancer cells. Your child will be treated with the above checked drugs, with your informed consent.

With my "informed consent"—I hardly see a choice involved as I take a deep breath to ease the tightness in my stomach and brush aside angry tears. I somehow know this list of power-packed drugs will not be powerful enough to produce a cure. They are only a means of buying time.

Impulsively I blurt out, "But what happens when you've gone

through this list? What happens when, even through rotation, to lessen the chance of leukemic cells becoming resistant to the drugs, they finally *do* become resistant? What are you going to do then? Don't answer. I don't really want to know." The gaze of Dr. Hays's eyes tells me the answer. But somewhere, in some lab, there's a scientist tirelessly perfecting *the* drug, *the* method of treatment, Kim will need and be ready for when this list is finis. *There's got to be!*

How can hope be mixed up with so many emotional opposites? That word always seems to carry a backlash now: hope-dread, hope-despair, hope-fear, hope-panic. God, will it ever be just *hope* again? We've been thrown off balance and occupy only one end of this traumatic, emotional seesaw. The erratic bumps of ups and downs have just begun.

When the lab report of Kim's blood tests comes in, Dr. Hays writes out the needed medication and dosage on a prescription slip and gives it to me. I take it downstairs to the pharmacy. This becomes regular routine. Waiting for the medication, I soon memorize the slowly changing displays in the glass counter fronting the pharmacy: a ship collection, a stamp collection, then a coin collection. While leaning against the corner wall, my fingers unconsciously tend to tap on the top of the glass counter. Then I know it is time to do something else, so I generally walk across to the volunteer gift shop that faces the pharmacy. In three years I memorize their inventory, but get tired of having to say, "No, thanks. I'm just looking," so many times. Finally my name is called, and I quickly turn to accept a very precious brown envelope—an envelope that contains vials and tablets of hope. I hurry back to the clinic, with the determined energy of fresh troops bringing reinforcements to the beleaguered front lines of battle.

And so each drug begins taking its turn at bat in Kim's system and in our hearts. How many innings will we play? Is there

enough equipment? We can't strike out! We've got to win! Jim
and I feel so exasperatingly desperate. Is this *all* that can be done?
Are we following the best possible course of treatment? Are we
in the best possible place for Kim to be treated? Does some other
hospital, in some other city, have newer drugs, better ways of
treatment? Have we trusted our only daughter's life to the very
best medical personnel in the treatment of childhood leukemia?
We're so ignorant of calamitous diseases! It's always been something that happens in someone else's family! "Oh, that I knew
where to find God—that I could go to his throne and talk with
him there" (Job 23:3).

We place a call to Dr. Earl Brewer, at Texas Children's Hospital, in Houston. Dr. Brewer was Kim's pediatrician in Wharton,
Texas, where she was born on March 13, 1961. He began practicing in Houston soon after our move there and so continued to
be our doctor for Jame and Kim. We had always thought very
highly of him as a friend and doctor, one whom we felt free to
call at any time.

It had been four years, but he remembers and is shocked to
hear of Kim's illness and the diagnosis. "You can bring her here
if you like, but I'd stay there, if I were you." Dr. Brewer goes on
to assure Jim and me of the reputation and reliability of Children's Hospital, in Denver, as a leading center for the treatment
of childhood cancers. If any new drug comes on the market, if
any new treatment proves successful, all the cancer-treatment
centers will receive whatever is available at relatively the same
time.

We decide to stay where we are. I think of Mary Jo. I think of
Dr. Hays. Beyond a doubt, I know we have made the right decision.

And so we wholeheartedly allow our lives and the life of our
child to become entrusted to the Oncology Clinic of Children's
Hospital, Denver, Colorado.

Like other departments of philosophy, medicine began with an age of wonder. The accidents of disease and the features of death aroused surprise and stimulated interest, and a beginning was made when man first asked in astonishment, "Why should these things be?"

SIR WILLIAM OSLER

4

The Search for Remission

IT IS TIME FOR A SHOWDOWN. Kim is scheduled for a bone-marrow test, the first since the onslaught of chemotherapy against
this indiscriminate enemy within.

In order to obtain the bone-marrow sample, a long hollow
needle is inserted into an area of active marrow production in the
hip bone. The needle is actually two parts: a hollow tube and a
solid plug to make it strong enough to get into a bone. Once inserted, the plug is pulled out, and the hollow tube left in place.
Then marrow is suctioned out through a syringe. Through the
use of special dyes, the physician can see the leukemic cells in
the sample. This procedure, called a bone-marrow aspiration, is
the most accurate course for following the disease. The proper
medication and dosages for the next month or so are prescribed
according to its evaluation. It is a time of anxious "what ifs?"
When Dr. Hays studies that slide under the microscope, what
will she see?

The goal we are shooting for is remission. To a leukemic patient, the word *remission* is a magic word, synonymous with hope.
To be told one is in remission is like slamming on the brakes at
the eroded edge of a dangerous precipice and having them hold
securely. Remission means a chance to snub our noses

at fate! And only the results of a bone-marrow test can tell us if that goal is attainable.

Jim comes from his office, to the waiting room of the oncology clinic. As we sit on the couch, our shoulders touch, balancing the load of anxiety pressing upon us. Kim has already gone to a treatment room.

A chilling, gut fear keeps us too restless for conversation. It's the sort of feeling that always comes with waiting—that horrible, draining expenditure of time.

Suddenly, over the audio of a TV game show, we hear an agonizing scream. Oh, God, it's my baby! Her scream pierces my soul with pain.

"I'll get some coffee." Jim walks quickly toward the elevator. My head falls to my knees, and I cover my ears.

God Almighty, please help my baby! Be with her. Pain is a brand-new acquaintance, too soon a part of her life. We're beyond Band-Aids on skinned knees and, "Let mommy kiss it better." Give her the strength to endure searing, grown-up pain without losing the exuberant joy of youth.

Dr. Hays comes into the waiting room. "Mrs. Jameson, you and Mr. Jameson can see Kim now, while we study the bone-marrow slide. I'm sorry it had to be so painful, but she really did quite well."

Jim comes back from the coffee shop, and we follow Dr. Hays through a wide, yellow door that has a torn-out coloring-book picture of Sleeping Beauty Scotch-taped over the window.

Kim is lying on her stomach, midst the wrinkled, protective sheets of the examining table. Her elbows are propped up and fists of wadded tissues support a tearstained face. I reach out for my child, wanting to gather her disturbed body in my arms and run away. She dissolves in tears.

Since Dr. Hays also did a spinal tap, Kim has to remain still for at least an hour. This lessens the chances of headache. Through this procedure (also called lumbar puncture) medicine is put into the cerebrospinal fluid (CSF). Leukemic blasts have a tendency to hide in the CSF. Because the CSF does not mix well with blood, medicines carried through the bloodstream are ineffective. A two-part needle is used, similar to one used in bone-marrow aspirations. It is inserted into the space in the spinal cord containing the CSF. After measuring the CSF pressure, methotrexate is put in. A study of the extracted cells is made under a microscope. If there are any blasts, they can be seen, and the doctors can find out if the leukemia has spread to the central nervous system and whether or not the treatment is working.

I sit in a small, wooden, child's chair and cradle Kim's perspiring face as she tries to tell us how much it hurt. Jim dampens his handkerchief, to wipe her face.

Mary Jo tries to ease the tension with light conversation. "Kim, do you still have your buckeye?"

"Of course." Slowly Kim unfolds her clenched fingers to reveal the buckeye in her wet palm. "You don't think I would be without it in a place like this, do you?"

Mary Jo tells us how Kim tried to explain the significance of having a Texas buckeye in her hand. Kim winks at me and rolls her eyes in the happy, secret expression of "we know something they don't."

Jim smiles.

I reach for that silly ol' buckeye and instinctively rub its shiny surface, my thoughts tumbling back over the years to the first time it became mine. Jim and I were high-school freshmen in Plainview, Texas. I played in the band, which was invited by the Cotton Bowl Committee to march during half-time activities of the Cotton Bowl game in Dallas on January 1, 1951. A spirit tradition was born when each member was given a dull, chestnut-like seed called a "buckeye." Only by continuous rubbing, in the ancient manner of Aladdin, could its surface take on the satiny sheen that supposedly would make our dreams and wishes come true.

In every uniform pocket, that cold New Year's Day in Dallas, Texas, was a shiny buckeye. Its tiny bulge reminded us "You *can* do it!" as we marched out from the goalposts in front of a sell-out crowd, proudly putting our small town on the map, through an impeccable performance.

Silly perhaps, maybe nonsense—but that buckeye remains a spirit-boosting symbol of "hang in there" and "you can do it."

I quickly learn that an element of humor is necessary in order for Kim to endure the harsh experiences of pain. Unfortunately this is sometimes interpreted as too much flippancy for a Christian.

"If I did not laugh, I should die" (Abraham Lincoln). To me Christianity has always meant response. I was always bursting at the seams, melting in the explosive, brilliant colors of life, as I believe God intended. "Don't just talk about God's love—*show me!*" That's what I try to do. I don't see anything sad about being a Christian. It is the happiest decision I ever made, and humor only adds depth and dimension to its meaning.

God surely has a sense of humor. How else could He have zonked the rhinoceros with that preposterous horn on his snout? or stretched out a long, curious neck on the giraffe? or curled the tail of a contented, mud-soaked pig? and done it all with a purpose, to boot! The curiosities of creation could not have been flukes. They were carefully planned and executed, and I believe, with a sense of humor!

"Man is distinguished from all other creatures by the faculty of laughter" (Joseph Addison).

"I have never understood why it should be considered derogatory to the Creator to suppose that he has a sense of humor" (William R. Inge).

To me, constant dejection and show of dispirit spell defeat. I want to see red! The color of fight—not the white flag of surrender! Aside from the power of prayer, my only other ammunition is a sense of humor. I pity those who cannot understand.

I put the buckeye back in my purse, for the time being.

Jim and I can see the bandaged area at the base of Kim's spine, between the bottom of her T-shirt and the top of her Levis. The very thought of Kim going through this regularly is unbearable. Yet it becomes a reality and is never easy.

The door opens, and Dr. Hays comes in. Her face is glowing. "Good news. Kim is in remission! The tests show no evidence of increased lymphoid blast cells. She is responding to the chemotherapy, just as we had hoped. You're very lucky, Kim! That first remission is very important!"

We are all weak with relief and joy. Thank You, God, thank You! Oh, *remission,* you are such a beautiful word! I am insane with hope, euphoric with relief.

Although Kim is exhausted and nauseous, the ride home is exhilarating. Our spirits soar on the tail of the rising kite of hope! At last we've caught the breeze of remission—up, up, and away! Fly! I shake off the knowledge that remission means a temporary arrest and has an opposite: relapse.

In the days ahead, Kim becomes herself again. Except for the irritating side effects of the antileukemic drugs, she is feeling great! Her personality begins to sparkle once more, as she runs to get on the busy carousel of preteen years.

My calendar fills with notations on drug dosages, between regular hospital appointments and blood tests: When tapering, divide prednisone in half every two days. Eight tablets of methotrexate on Tuesday and Friday. I don't really have to worry about keeping it all straight. Kim never forgets. Little do I realize this first remission is only the beginning of a savage emotional seesaw.

Death seems remote now. The mountains viewed from my kitchen window no longer look threatening. Their snow-capped peaks rise majestically toward the crisp, blue Colorado sky— reaching, telling me, reminding me, Look up! God is still in control and is powerful enough and resourceful enough to bring good out of any situation. I must be patient. Trust Him. Yes, I really believe I would have failed to recognize the significance of the beauty of those mountain peaks, if I had not seen them first from the depths of this deep, dark valley.

God, I'm just now getting to know You, aren't I? All these years, I only thought I knew You. It was more an acquaintance-ship than a friendship. An acquaintance, one is aware of. A friend, one knows. An ideal, one strives and works for. A Father, one trusts and lives for. A Saviour, one loves, in total, individual commitment. Dear God, my Friend, Father, Saviour—how complex are Your ways, as I ponder my own existence in the enormity of Your universe. "When I consider thy heavens, the work of thy fingers, the moon and the stars, which thou hast ordained; What is man, that thou art mindful of him? . . ." (Psalms 8:3, 4 KJV).

I do feel Your presence in this faith-snatching situation, God. I feel Your quiet prodding of, "Trust Me, trust Me, despair is presumptuous." But it is so hard to "let go, and let God" when I've been used to leading, instead of following.

Thank You for the light of remission we've reached around the bend of this dark path of tragedy. And even if the light should dim and plunge us into darkness once more, give us the strength to keep plodding. Help me to develop hind's feet, if the path narrows and becomes more treacherous. I think I'm going to need them. Help me somehow to understand what's happening.

Days dissolve into accelerating weeks, as hospital appointments and chemotherapy treatments become part of a normal, hectic, happy family schedule. Despondency is put on the back burner. My old clownish personality emerges.

Hey, we're laughing again! Hello CO-LO-RA-DO! We ain't down yet! Let the sunshine in. Hold it, clouds! It feels so warm and safe. The shimmering gold of the aspen, a winter wonderland with the first snowfall—how beautiful. How simply wonderful to be alive! O God, how great Thou art! Football games,

piano lessons, camping trips, ice skating, skiing attempts—we're back to normal! Everything's okay, isn't it? Could a mistake in the diagnosis possibly have been made? Have our prayers already been answered? Breathing deeply of invincibility brings renewed strength to challenge our fate.

Now that Kim is in remission, we are confronted with the necessity of radiation therapy. It is a snap back to reality. The membranes of the skull are vulnerable hiding places for lurking leukemic cells waiting to strike again. This sanctuary must be eradicated.

Because antileukemic drugs do not pass the so-called blood-brain barrier, it is possible for the central nervous system (CNS) to be invaded by leukemic cells, during a period of complete remission. Prevention of this attack is a major area of clinical research. At present, radiotherapy is the ace in the hole.

I begin to resent having to plan for radiotherapy. I even hate to take Kim back to the hospital to get her finger pricked for blood tests. Besides, she complains, pulling off the Band-Aid ruins a careful manicure!

She's too busy living to be reminded she's dying—maybe.

5

Meeting the Monster

> Went to the hospital and they took a blood sample and gave
> me some medicine. But now they're talking about giving me
> radiation in my head! I'm really scared. I don't know what to
> think!

NEITHER DO I. I absorbed the knowledge of this precautionary
method of treatment in the initial shock. Now it surfaces again.
Radiation: It's even an awesome word to say—a word of fear, of
things unknown. Now it concerns me and my child. I feel like an
idiot even thinking this, but I secretly wonder if it might damage
her brain. Oh, God, there's so much to learn and be knowledge-
able about. Where have I been all my life?

Arrangements are made for Kim to begin radiation treatments
at Presbyterian Medical Center. She is to receive radiation every
day, for the next three weeks. I schedule appointments so she
will miss as few classes as possible.

Once again I reach for my tattered city map of Denver, under
the front seat of my car, to locate another hospital. The streets in
this medical center are too narrow for two-way traffic! Cars are
honking at me to move on, and I haven't the slightest idea where
to go! Spotting the hospital parking lot, I tell Kim, "Shut your

eyes and hold your breath, podner. We're headin' for open pasture!"

She grins and lays her head back. "Mom, I really don't feel good enough for you to have another fender bender!"

Finally, here it is. A step on the entry mat, and the electric door of Presbyterian Medical Center slides open for the first of many times. It's a giant step indeed.

At the information desk, a volunteer gives us directions to the radiation-therapy department. They have colored dots on the floor, to direct people to the various departments. Kim and I exchange grins as we're told to follow the yellow dots.

"Follow the yellow brick road—ta dum—follow the yellow brick road—ta dum———" We start humming that familiar tune, stepping on as many dots as we can, very discreetly, of course, and snickering like a couple of little kids! It is a natural response, after having spent years turning most any experience into a game. Though I know it somehow must continue as an invaluable morale booster, playing games proves to be a continuing challenge of intense effort.

Kim is laughing. "Mother, they're going to put a net over you, one of these days!"

Eureka! Here's the door. I'm supposed to ask to see Dr. R. L. Penniman. We practice saying his name. Kim is so afraid I'm going to slip and say Dr. Feen-a-mint! We sit in the only two empty chairs in the waiting room.

We're not laughing anymore. I feel like the rubber scrap of a popped balloon, as I glance at the people sitting around us. Oh, dear God, we've got to be in the wrong place! A man sitting across from us has no hair at all. His glowing scalp is reddish and splotchy, with ink markings across the center. Skin drapes loosely over his skull. Next to him is a lady, actually quite young looking, with only a few wispy strands of auburn hair on one side of her head. Her right ear is swollen and covered with red, crusty-looking sores. She's busy knitting.

My eyes rivet the floor. I don't want to see any more! Kim's saddle oxfords are still, but I detect a tremor inside those white knee socks. "C'mon, Kim. Let's go get a Coke." She grasps my hand as we step quickly out into the hall.

"Oh, mother, I'm so scared!" she whispers in a shaky voice. "They look so awful!" She touches the ends of her pigtails. "Am *I* going to look horrible?"

I glance at her desperate face, my fingers scrambling for change for the cold-drink machine. "Don't be afraid, baby. God is with us." God, I'm scared, too!

We finish our Cokes out in the hall. When Kim's name is called, we walk briskly back through the waiting room. I wonder if the waiting will get any easier. It doesn't. Time spent in the waiting room remains consistently depressing, like sitting in an atmosphere of falling gray silk.

What's the matter with you, brain? I'm only getting messages to run, scream, faint! Don't you realize that Kim's reaction will depend a great deal upon your own? C'mon now, walk, legs! Loosen grip on Kim's hand. Listen to what's being said. Breathe calmly, as though this were not the first time you've seen life in battle with death. Oh, God, it *is* the first time!

After Kim's examination, the procedures to be followed for the next few weeks are explained. We turn toward a door at the end of the hall, as the tour continues.

I hear a humming sound. The big door opens slowly, quietly. We step inside.

"And *this* is LINAC, a four-million-volt linear accelerator." I feel as if we're being introduced to King Kong, as my gaze follows the awesome lines of this monstrous-looking machine. LINAC is the first machine of the linear-accelerator type to be installed in this area. The phrase "linear accelerator" refers to the principle on which this machine operates. The heart of the machine is a twelve-inch long accelerator tube in which electrons are accelerated, in a linear manner, to a total energy of four million volts. These high-energy electrons are made to strike a water-cooled metal target and thus produce high energy X rays. These X rays are similar to the radiation produced by cobalt units, but are of higher energy and of greater intensity. The force which accelerates the electrons down the tube is bursts of very high frequency radio waves.

ᛐ The shock waves of the technicality of this information and how it relates to us stuns my mind.

I'm staring at the technologist who is talking, but my ears are refusing to hear. Fear is closing the door on my ability to understand. All I receive is the fact that Kim will be sealed off in that room, all alone, lying on a slab, with the heart of that overpowering machine hovering above her head! Don't let her be afraid, Lord. Give my baby courage.

"Do you have any questions?" I shake my head mechanically and murmur a no. But I'm smothering under an avalanche of information I don't understand. Kim stares quietly at the floor, her face void of expression.

"Well then, why don't we step outside, and I'll explain to Kim what we want her to do. Then we'll watch her receive the treatment, on closed-circuit television."

Jim is at the door, when we turn to leave the room. I want to run into the comfort of his arms, like a scared, lost child. But I don't dare show any emotion. He puts his arm around Kim's shoulders as the technician introduces LINAC to him.

Kim is placed on the table and shown the position in which she must remain motionless. The heavy door closes slowly behind us as we walk out of the room. To the right is the 4MV LINAC control panel. Our eyes are fixed on the tiny black and white TV screen, overhead, as Kim's still figure, lying on that table, comes in view.

Kim is given instructions over the intercom, and the procedure is begun. I hold my breath. My eyes are glued to that screen, my mind and heart silently pleading with that machine. Please

LINAC, don't be the monster you appear to be! Work for us, be our friend. That's our Kim you've got under your control in there.

"That's it, Mr. and Mrs. Jameson. It's all over. This is the procedure that will be followed every day for the next three weeks. Most of the time, as you can see, is spent in preparation. Kim did everything beautifully."

Jim and I wait outside as Kim is helped off the table and answers some questions. She walks haltingly toward us, looking quite relieved. "I really didn't feel anything, mother, but I'm sure glad it's over—the first time at least." So are we. Jim walks us to the car before going back to work.

Reluctantly, Kim accepts this new routine. The days are long and tiring though, now that school has started. She begins dreading the long trips downtown, the interruption in her struggle to break in a new school. During the second week of treatments Kim begins referring to the LINAC as the Monster.

She hates the Monster, not for what it can or cannot do for her well-being, but because she knows as soon as the treatments are over her hair will begin falling out.

> Didn't feel good enough to go to school, so mother went and got my assignments. I felt a little better, after resting. Started radiation treatments at Presbyterian Hospital. I didn't feel it, but it was scary. We have to go back tomorrow.

6

Walk by Faith

MY DEAR POSTMAN, do you possibly realize what an important job you have, stopping at our house every day? Do you realize the significance of those letters you so casually place in our mailbox?

Kim saves every card and letter, in shoe boxes under her bed. Those boxes become symbols of love and hope.

Every Wednesday a bulging envelope comes from Willow Meadows Baptist Church, in Houston, containing dozens of prayer-time cards. Many are written by people we never met, but who are just as concerned as our friends who know and care for us. So often a long-distance phone call or a card bearing the signatures of dozens of friends enables Kim to recover enough spirit and determination to meet the trials of another day.

Dear Kim,

Hi! How have you been? What have you been doing? Guess what? I made cheerleader for Oaklawn Junior High! I was so happy! I know you would have made it, too, if you still lived here. I miss you so very much! I still have your last year's picture. I bet you're even prettier now! Do you still play the piano? Have you won any more talent-show trophies? Please write back soon, and take

care of yourself. Kim, you always tell me to *smile,* so *smile!*
God loves *everybody!*

Friends always,
CINDY REMBERT

Dear Kim,

It was great to get your beautiful letter. As you guessed, the weather here in Pennsylvania is getting cold, and all the leaves are gone.

I'm sure you will find a piano teacher that you will like in Colorado. In the meantime, keep working with your mom. She is a great, talented lady. Keep me posted on how you are feeling. I enjoy your letters!

Love,
MR. CRAMER

Dear Kim,

I hope those radiation treatments help you. I'm sure they will, and maybe those headaches will be over with soon, too. Don't worry about me telling everybody about your hair, 'cause I won't.

Friends always,
RACHEL MARTIN

Dear Kim,

"Along the way take time to smell the flowers. Flowers are a blooming festival of life. Let no flower go unseen. Bloom where you are planted." Ya like that? I do.

Guess what! My mother is going to have a baby!

I just want to wish you a merry Christmas, Kim. I miss you so much, you were the best friend I ever had.

Your friend always,
DENA DUMONT

Dear Kim,

Hi! I am Dr. Dobson's secretary, Robye Bryan. I guess you call him Papa, though. It wouldn't make sense to call your granddad Dr. Dobson! What I really wanted you to know is that you have been a blessing to my life, even though I've never met you. You're very brave, and I know it is because you have Jesus Christ in your heart and life. I hope you will continue in your faith and cheerful attitude. There are a lot of people, here in Brownwood, who are praying for you. I love your grandparents very much, but don't tell them until I get out of their classes here at Howard Payne! They might think I was trying to get an A! Take care, Kim, and remember what you told your grandfather once in a letter, "God loves you . . . and I love you." May God bless you!

In His love,
ROBYE BRYAN

When I got back from school, the biggest package I've ever seen was waiting for me! My best friend in New Orleans, Debbie Ledet, had sent it from all my friends at the First Baptist Church. I was so surprised! Mom helped me open it, and she was as excited as me! It was a great, big, stuffed dog, as tall as me! Oh, I'm so *happy!* I'm going to name it Saint Charles.

It's late, but I'm determined to finish straightening the shelves in my bedroom closet, before going to bed. Kim calls out to me and starts to cry as I walk into her darkened room. She pulls back the patchwork quilt, and I lie down beside her. The Victorian charm of her canopy bed always provides a special warmth and closeness as we share hopes, reveal secrets, and discuss disappointments. It's our favorite place for "girl talk."

"Oh, mom, why does something so bad have to happen to me when I'm so far away from all my friends? They won't care, even if I do get bald. I'll be such an oddball here; *nobody* will like me! They just would never understand. Mother, we're even Christians; how can such a thing happen to us? Everything used to be so good. Is God mad at us or something? I just don't understand. I'm more normal than most people!"

I hold her close, as her body heaves with sobs. My God, my God, I don't understand, either. You've hurled a storm at us, and we're struggling against the wind. It's hard to keep looking up, when the magnet of despair is pulling us into a sea of despondency. My feet are wet, and I don't like it. The billowing waves of problems and fears are drawing my eyes away from You, my source of power. And it *can* happen, just as it did to Simon Peter.

Save me, Lord. Doubt is causing me to sink. Fix my gaze upon You, that I might not falter. I'm concentrating on my weakness, instead of on Your strength. The fog of doubt is so dense I can't see You, Lord! Do *You* see *us?* ". . Lo, I am with you always . . ." (Matthew 28:20 KJV). Give me the patience to let my faith work and not drown out Your "still small voice" with my screaming, "Why don't You *do* something!" This fog challenges my faith. I will either fall in defeat, and You will be obscured, or I will rise to meet it, and You will be revealed. I accept the challenge!

> I would rather walk in the dark with Him
> Than walk alone in light.
> I would rather walk by faith in Him
> Than walk alone by sight.

It's going to be a long walk, Kim, but we're not alone. Good night, my darling. Good night, Saint Charles.

7

The Love of Friends

KIM'S COUNSELOR at Newton Junior High School, Dorothy Buckley, becomes her ally, confidante, and advisor through many
embarrassing and difficult situations. We work out excuses and
pass slips so Kim's absences will be less noticeable to her classmates. Her greatest fear is someone finding out something is the
matter with her. Her teachers are helpful and cooperative with
make-up work and respect her wishes to not be treated differently. They keep her secret so well that Kim's condition becomes known only gradually, and only when Kim is just too
weary to think up more excuses.

I watch anxiously, from her upstairs bedroom window, as she
walks slowly but determinedly toward a group of kids she
doesn't know, standing at the bus stop down the street from our
house. I kneel by her bed and weep and pray for a long time.

Some days Kim needs a transfusion or some other method of
tedious chemotherapy. Then I rush her back to school in time for
the next class. She hates to be absent, no matter how she feels.
When she wants to go home, I know her energy is completely
drained. Her school books are always with her. She tries hard not
to get behind.

Most of the time, her teachers are unaware of any painful ordeal Kim has already undergone that day. It is like leading two

lives. She is fighting to survive and at the same time is calmly being "like everybody else." The charade ends in the blessed privacy of our home.

> **September 25** I was having real bad headaches, so I couldn't go to school. This medicine sure doesn't seem to be helping!

> **September 27** I went to school, but my head was pounding before first hour was over, and I had to call mom to come get me. Slept until it was time for radiation. Dad met us at Presbyterian. Afterwards we went to the last part of Jame's football game. Arapahoe won! Jame was real happy, and so were we. I was having such bad headaches by the time we got home that I didn't feel like doing much.

Kim seeks to make her own way without what she calls mushy sympathy. She is lonely and wants desperately to make friends. But she wants kids to like her for *herself*. Leukemia is not to be used as a free pass.

Kim is blessed with a happy, outgoing, fun-loving personality. Moving so often, we joke about her casing the new neighborhood and seeing how quickly she can return, surrounded by new friends. Getting acquainted and involved in a new community has never before been a problem. Now it is.

That bubbly daughter of mine is a natural leader, joiner, and participant. Now all of that is being challenged. Will those qualities still manage to surface? Will she make it?

I remember that anxious morning, only three weeks before—September 4—as she left the house to begin junior high. She left with tremendous emotional and physical pressures, too heavy for her age, concealed behind a nervous smile.

> **September 28** Tried to go to school and made it up until English class, and my headache got so bad I had to call mom to come get me again. It was rainy and cold, but we went on

down to Children's. Dr. Hays gave me some medicine. I sure do hope it works.

September 29 I got scared about my disease during church. I don't feel as if I know everything about it! After church we drove out to Lookout Mountain and saw Buffalo Bill's grave. That was fun.

It dawns on me that time is not going to heal Kim's wounded spirits. As a family, we can do just so much. She becomes depressed, thinking about her old friends and the good times we left. She needs a new friend, one she can feel close to, who can activate her will to get it going again.

That incredible gift of friendship. How fortunate we have been to possess so much of it. It was a treasure taken for granted—not anymore. I find myself clinging to the memory of each one. Though far away, our friends seem to grow around us, like a supporting vine. And yet we feel so alone! How I long to see them! Why did such a calamity come to us in the midst of a move, so far away from people and places that could bring such comfort just by being there. To be surrounded by friends, when one's soul is chilled, is to be warmed by a blanket of love. Dear God, I'm so cold.

October 1 Got up and ready for school. Made it through the whole day without having to go home! Mom picked me up right after school, since we had to go to the hospital for radiation. When we got there, we had to wait for almost an hour. I hate to have to wait there.

October 2 I made it through the whole day without getting a *bad* headache. When we got back from the hospital, Jame was home from school, sick with a virus. Now we're both sick! I wish I just had a virus.

October 4 Went to school, but had to get out right after art class, to go to Children's Hospital. I had a blood test, and then

Dr. Hays talked to mom and me. I have to go back Monday
for a spinal tap—*ugh!* I wish I could find a best friend. I get so
depressed.

The school bus screeches to a stop at the corner. Oh, my gosh,
where has this day gone? There seems to be so little time to work
on the house, without interruptions. Daisy, our basset hound,
hurries to the front door, waiting for it to burst open, her tail
wagging like a windshield wiper at high speed. She doesn't have
long to wait.

"Mom," the door slams shut, "you've got to meet the neatest
girl! Her name is Pam Bergin, and I just love her and want to be
best friends with her more than anything! She wants me to come
over tomorrow, after school. I could ride the bus with her to her
house. Could you pick me up, so you could meet her and her
mom? She already has a best friend, but I think she likes me well
enough to have two best friends! I hope so."

And so Pam Bergin enters our lives. Thank You, God. In the
next three years, Pam will be all the warm friendships Kim
misses rolled into one: a tangible friend Kim can play with, cry
with, laugh with, study with—just be with—every day. Kim
begins to have a feeling of standing a chance in the world of her
peers, again. Between Pam and the supportive correspondence of
her best friend in New Orleans, Debbie Ledet, Kim endures
many intolerable experiences. The friendship of these two girls is
as important to her well-being as any medicine could possibly be.

The phone starts to ring again, followed by a split-second "I'll
get it!"

I begin finding notes in sweater pockets again, while sorting
the wash:

"Hi, Kim, Pam here. Remember me? If you try to call me
tonight, I won't be home. I'll be baby-sitting.

I don't know why Keely has to move. I cried for a whole evening, when I found out. She's the best friend I've got. Do you think we could be pretty good friends? I hope so. Right now you're my second-best friend.

Have you ever had a real neat guy for a boyfriend? When's your birthday? What kind of animals do you have in your family? Do you babysit? Are you and your family close?

Oh, I've run out of paper. Boy, does paper fly—ha-ha-ha!

P<small>AM</small> B.

It's the beginning of a beautiful friendship. Pam becomes a special part of our family, and we love her as a daughter. The ice of loneliness is finally starting to crack. Pam Bergin—a timely prescription for Kim that only God could have filled.

Dear Debbie,

I hope you will please forgive me for not writing, but I've been busy up to my ears with school and church— and I guess pretty lazy, too! When my hair grows back, I want it to grow back like your new haircut! My hair is starting to come out real badly now. I'll probably look like a little boy with a burr, pretty soon.

The mountains are so pretty. I love to go driving in them. It seems as if you are so far away from everything and everybody. I have to have a spinal tap and bone-marrow pretty soon. I am so scared. It's probably just built up in my mind so much that I believe it. But I can't think of anything else that hurts more.

How 'bout this: "If Christ came today, what would your tomorrow be like?" I read that somewhere.

Give everyone down there in ol' New Orleans my love.
Hope we can come to see y'all next Mardi Gras—cross
your fingers!

Luv 'ya
Friends Forever
Kɪᴍ

"A friend in need," my neighbor said to me;
"A friend in need, is what I mean to be.
In time of trouble I will come to you,
And in the hour of need you'll find me true."

I thought a bit, then took him by the hand;
"My friend," I said, "you do not understand
The inner meaning of that simple rhyme;
A friend is what the heart needs all the time."

Aᴜᴛʜᴏʀ Uɴᴋɴᴏᴡɴ

No price tag can be put on the worth of true friendship. It is a
seed to be planted, nurtured, cultivated, harvested. It is that plus
quality that gives real meaning to the Christian concept of the
worth of every person. It is a gift from God to the world. "I
would not live without the love of my friends" (John Keats).

8

Facing the Changes

By MID-OCTOBER the reality of Kim actually losing her hair has to be faced. I pretend not to notice how thin it is getting. I try to overlook the hairbrush full of long, static-crazed hair in the bathroom each morning and the long, wandering hairs clinging to her pillowcase. I try so hard to not see, but I do see! And a nauseating chill comes over me, each time.

Oh, God, please don't let her look any different! I couldn't stand that! We can cope, as long as we can't see! I have been so concerned with how Kim's body reacts to the antileukemic drugs, that I have not come to terms with any possible outward changes. Now I must.

Dr. Hays suggests I have Kim's hair cut shorter, at least shoulder length, so the loss won't be so emotionally severe. Reluctantly, I make an appointment. Kim doesn't want to forget how long her hair has been, so I snap her picture in the parking lot before we go in. I feel as if I am leading her to a slaughterhouse.

This is such an ordeal to go through, especially not knowing the beautician and the beautician not knowing our situation. We endure small, senseless chatter: "You know, dear, you may be starting a new style. Most of the girls your age *want* their hair nice and long, like yours is now." Kim manages a shrug of the shoulders and rigidly clamps her fingers over the ends of the chair arms. Snap, the plastic cape is fastened and smoothed over her taut body. I walk over to an empty chair, behind a plastic rubber plant, and welcome the relief of sitting down. I pick up a magazine. But my concentration is hardly on Hollywood gossip. My perspiring hands freeze to the pages, as I stare over the top of that magazine, watching in calm horror, as clump after clump of Kim's dark brown hair falls and scatters to the floor. We are both having our insides cut to pieces, as the scissors go snip, snip, snip.

After that ordeal is over, we have to face buying a wig. It is important that Kim has one before it is needed, to give her time to get used to the idea.

"But mother, kids don't wear wigs! What if it falls off? Oh, Mother I just can't! I'll look so ugly and different. I don't care if I just die right now!"

In the car she puts her head in my lap, under the steering wheel, and cries softly all the way into town.

Pardon me, God, but I've got to ask again: why? Looks are so important to girls at this age. They're so caught up in the changes their bodies are going through, as traces of the little girl disappear with each passing day. It's hard enough just battling what's going on inside! Oh, how I hurt for my child. Help us, God, everything seems beyond control!

Kim grimaces and holds her breath as Dolly, the saleslady, tries on the first wig. "Now don't worry about how it looks," Dolly says, shifting the cap and tucking Kim's own diminishing locks underneath. "I'm just trying to get a good fit. When we decide on one, I'll shape it, comb it, and cut it to make it look just like you."

Kim's eyes brim with tears. Her fingers tightly close around the arms of the chair.

God, it *does* look awful! And Kim knows it! She looks as if she were being made up to play the mother in a child's play.

I feel like throwing up, collapsing my rubbery knees to the

floor and dissolving into one big heap of heartaches. But I smile and tell Kim to try to be patient. Dolly tries others on her.

Finally, voice trembling, Kim says, "Mom, what do you think?"

"Well, Kim, I like that one. I really do. I believe it is one we can work with. It's youthful, exactly the same color as your own." Dolly had cut a longer wig into a pageboy style that could be worn with different headbands.

"You're not just saying that?"

"No, honey, let's take that one. You'll have plenty of time to work with it and get it looking even more natural."

A mink-wrapped, matronly customer strolls into the wig department, with an air of owning the store. She passes by Kim's chair as Dolly is finishing her wig and comments in a low, biting voice, "Well, I declare, the younger generation is certainly in a big hurry to look grown up." I pray that Kim didn't hear, as I control my surging anger. Dolly lets Kim's chair down, and we hurriedly gather our things to leave. We are just beginning to know the cruelty of words spoken in thoughtless ignorance.

We drive home in silence. Kim lays her head down after a while, muffling sobs in my lap. The wig box lies unopened on the floor. I pat her shoulders gently and reach for her hand. A carload of teenage girls pulls up beside our car, at a red light. Their gaiety and laughter and preoccupation with their own little world drifts eerily to us. The long, blond hair of the girl driving blows tauntingly in the breeze—two cars side-by-side, with youth at its best riding in both. But knowledge of the value of life, learned through struggle, is a passenger in one. And knowledge of the joys of life, flippantly taken for granted, is a passenger in the other. They are cars on different paths to a common destination.

And so begin hours in the bathroom, with the door shut, as Kim and her wig become acquainted. The emotional outbursts and rebellious tirades coming from behind that closed door scathe my heart: the sound of a comb breaking in the sink, a brush thrown to the floor, wrenching sobs of despair.

It's enough. I open the door. "Kim, let me help you, honey. Let's try again."

"Oh, Mother, I hate it. I hate it!" She throws the wig to the floor. "Mom, I'm going to be so ugly. What'll I do?"

God, help us. Though she's as tall as me, I gather her into my arms as I used to do when she was little. But now her sorrows match and mingle with my own. I can no longer say, "There, now, everything is going to be all right."

This one psychological, as well as physical, problem will be the hardest to endure—one that is never overcome and always makes Kim vulnerable to new hurts.

Kim barely combs her hair now, doing all she can to keep it from falling out. But more and more of her scalp begins to show. Her eyes look so large to me, then I realize it is because I can clearly see the shape of her whole head! What a devastating blow. It also affects Jim and Jame, but we never never speak of it, pretending not to notice, in order to ease her self-consciousness.

The day comes when she either has to wear the wig or stay home from school the next day. Kim calls Pam to come over and help. From the kitchen, I hear the opening and shutting of bedroom and bathroom doors, upstairs, as the girls go back and forth. The record player is going, and I even hear an occasional outburst of laughter! God, thank You for Pam!

It isn't long before they bound downstairs, ready to give an improvised style show. I relax, thoroughly enjoying the change in atmosphere. Kim is ready for tomorrow. Bless you, Pam.

Kim gets up earlier than usual the next morning, to allow plenty of time to fix her wig. She wears it with a little handkerchief scarf tied to the back, underneath. I busy myself with breakfast dishes and making lunches, to keep my thoughts from wandering too freely. I need to draw something special on her lunch napkin today.

This is a custom that started when Jame was in first grade. By now, of course, he's outgrown cartoons and "thoughts for today" in his lunch sack. I still let him have it on his birthday, though, and on holidays. I fill the Frito bag with plastic foam and discreetly reseal it, put a plastic hard-boiled egg in a Baggie, and pour confetti over everything, before stapling the sack shut. Though my children would never admit it, they both thoroughly enjoy kooky Mom's sense of humor. The biggest howls of protest came on Saint Patrick's Day, when they poured green milk out of their Thermos bottles!

I spread out the paper napkin and reach for my pen. Quickly I sketch a stick-figure girl with a round face, hurrying out the front door of a house, empty-handed. Scrawling *whoops* in big letters, her feet draw up in a braking position. Then I draw her coming back out of the house, with a big smile on her face, a stylish hairdo, carrying books and a big satchel, marked *smiles,* with smiles spilling out and leaving a trail. A smiling sun, in the corner, whistles "Oh, You Beautiful Doll." A directional sign in a clump of grass reads, "Have a nice day!" I fold the napkin around two prednisone tablets and staple her lunch sack shut.

The doorbell rings. Daisy beats me to the front door. She gets so excited, thinking it surely means someone has come to play with her and pet her. What pleasure and comfort that lovable, silly-looking dog brings to us all.

Tammy and Ginger True are at the door, to walk to the bus stop with Kim. With books under her arm, Kim hurries into the kitchen, to pick up her lunch. "How do I look, mom? Is it okay? Are you sure? Are you absolutely positive the wig looks natural? Can you tell, I mean, if you didn't already know? Now tell me honestly!"

I give her a kiss on the cheek. The wig does look good; she is cute as ever. "You look absolutely ravishing, my dear! A padded bra couldn't keep a better secret! Just keep that chin up, look happy, and remember the secret word is *confidence!*" She gives me a peck on the cheek and rushes to the door. The girls leave in a flurry of conversation.

I shut the door and sit down on the bottom stair, reaching out to hug Daisy, as she waddles over. Bless this day, Lord. Thank You for it. Help Jim in his new job, as he balances those pressures with the ones at home. Help Jame today. Don't let me be blinded to his needs and hurts. He probably has more than I realize. And help Kim. You're the only one who can. Build up in her a reservoir of confidence and trust in You that will see her through this experience and others to follow. And please help me, Lord. Three people, and a dog, are depending on me to set the mood and pace of each day! But I'm a person, too, with needs for encouragement and inner strength of my own. So, when my family all go their separate ways, each morning, and the door shuts for the last time, gear me up for the pace of my day. Help me to someday, somehow, make sense out of what Paul said in First Thessalonians about giving thanks in all circumstances. That's really having faith in You, isn't it? Having the assurance that You are at work in this whole process of tragedy and being able to give thanks in the meantime. My faith has never really been stretched before, God. Forgive the creaking, rusty sounds of enlargement. And, by the way, thank You.

9

Lord, Keep Her Climbing

DESPITE THE PROBLEMS of headaches, upset stomachs, and losing her hair as the radiation treatments end, Kim is managing her life very well. She misses little school. Our lives somehow expand to take in these new adjustments.

> **October 28** Brrrrrrr, it's *cold!* Wore my wig to church. I worked on it all day yesterday and last night, but I still feel as if everybody is staring at me! I'm so scared it's going to fall off, and there's nothing to pin it to! Went to bed feeling kinda so-so.

I open the pantry door and stare at my kitchen calendar, hanging inside. Conflicting feelings of rising anticipation and lurking dread sweep over me. Holidays are coming up. It's only a few days before Halloween. A nostalgic longing for the carefree excitement of planning for Halloween, and all other holidays, overwhelms me. Such a fun time, its memory now carries an aching stigma.

Can I do it again? Kim is already talking about it. How can I psych myself up to carry on the traditions, started years ago, when the children were little, that make holidays so special in our family? And yet traditions seem more important now than ever before. In fact each day seems more important. Is it because an unvoiced question keeps surfacing in my mind, "Is this the last Halloween for Kim? Will this be her last Christmas? Will she have another birthday?" Oh, God, I don't know how to live for today; there's always been a tomorrow! I don't know how to shift gears from always to now!

Sometimes I feel like a clown, God, hiding a broken heart behind the makeup of a smiling face, compelled to keep up the show-must-go-on spirit, because others depend on my performance to keep going, themselves. This comic streak is no longer just a frivolous side of my personality; it is a valuable defense against melancholy and depression.

> **October 31** BOO! Tammy and I finally decided we'd go out
> with the trick-or-treaters for a while, but we went around the
> neighborhood first for UNICEF. Mother, as usual, scared all
> the kids to death, in her witch costume, but they loved it and
> kept coming back! It was so much fun.

Just recalling those fun, special days bring such pain now. I was making deposits into memory banks, to withdraw happiness from when Jame and Kim were grown and away from home. All the slides and picture albums are supposed to bring such pleasure in later years.

I never dreamed pleasant memories could also bring such haunting pain. My reserve is drained. How can I continue to make deposits, when the memories that are already there turn on me, reminding me of times that can never be again, making me question ever having the experience of happiness again, as each celebration is clouded by that haunting question, "Will this be the last?"

It is time to flip a page on my kitchen calendar: November—Thanksgiving.

November 6 Got to school, and the guy with a locker next to mine talked to me! He seems real nice! During fifth period Joan Quigley broke her arm in P.E. It was real bad. I felt so sorry for her, when I heard about it. But I doubt that it's as bad as having leukemia.

When I got home, mother was painting the fireplace from ugly green to white. Hope we can get things cleaned up enough to have a Thanksgiving dinner!

November 14 Watched *Brian's Song* on TV. I couldn't help crying. I went to bed real sad and thinkin'.

The incident I dread most happens to Kim the afternoon of November 21. Dorothy Buckley calls from school. Someone pulled off Kim's wig, in the hall, between classes.

"I'll be right there." I reach for the car keys and slam the back door in bitterness, thinking of all the pieces of shattered confidence I would somehow have to put back together.

When I pull in front of the school, Kim throws her books in the car. She falls across the seat, dissolving in tears of despair and humiliation. "Oh, mother, mother, it was just awful! I'm never going back to school again!"

I hug her and pull the car back into the lane of traffic. Help us, God! Help me to know how to comfort without letting my anger oversympathize. Give me the wisdom of patient control. We need the warmth of Your strength and compassion on this cold, distressing day. Tomorrow is Thanksgiving. Don't let us forget all we have to be thankful for, in spite of this dreadful incident!

At home Kim slings her wig on the floor and drops, sobbing, on the den couch. "Mother, it was just horrible! The hall was real noisy and crowded, as it always is between classes, and I was walking close to the lockers. Suddenly I felt my wig slip! I grabbed it at my shoulder and tried to hold it in place, with my head down, and ran for the rest room. The kids were hollering and laughing around me."

"I just sat down on the floor in the rest room and started shaking and crying and couldn't stop. A girl in one of my classes came in and asked me if I was sick, and I told her to please get Mrs. Buckley. I wasn't going back out in that hall until everyone was gone.

"What am I going to do, mom? How can I ever face going back? I feel as if the whole school is staring at me and hollering, 'Freak, freak, freak, that new girl is a bald freak!' My classes are getting harder, and I want to make friends and be like the other kids, but I'm just so tired of everything."

Gently I pull her limp, disillusioned body against my own. Though I can soothe and love, I am powerless to protect my child against the knocks and hurts of the world. The battleground on which leukemia is fought cannot be confined to the protective walls of a hospital clinic, or even to our home. Over her shoulder, my eyes glance around at the visible pains a house goes through before becoming a home. The half-painted walls are taking on character now—the character of a fortress.

"Kim, I would give anything to protect you from hurts like this, but I can't, not without isolating you. And I don't think you want that. But, with God's help, I believe we can build up enough strength to withstand and overcome them. It's a matter of not giving up when the battle gets tough. And each time you withstand one skirmish, you gain strength to withstand and conquer another. It's a reinforcement process that cannot take place unless you determine to stand up to the problem and meet it with all the control and courage you can muster." Kim does not answer.

"Oh, honey, it would be so easy for me to say, 'Stay home, Kim. We'll get a tutor, and you won't have to go back to school and risk being hurt and humiliated. . . .' "

We talk on the couch until it's time to get dinner.

I promise to get a wig liner, from Dolly, that will make her wig fit more securely. "Okay, babe?" Kim, my precious Kim, I love you so very much! "Look, why don't you take a nap, and then you can help me make the pies for tomorrow's dinner. It's Thanksgiving, remember?"

The phone rings as Kim slowly gets up. It's Mrs. Buckley, wanting to tell Kim again how sorry she is about the incident and urging her to come back to school Monday. I breathe a prayer of relief and thanks as I hear Kim say, "I'll try, Mrs. Buckley."

I listen to her climb the stairs to her room, each foot shifting slowly up the recently sanded steps as if lifting it required the greatest effort. But it's progress, dear God, it's *progress!* Keep her climbing!

I can no longer hold back my tears and bury my face in my apron. Oh, God, it's so unfair! How much can Kim take without her spirit being destroyed? Only through trials is real courage born. Is she going to need that much grown-up courage?

My only comfort is knowing You feel and hurt with us. And that is a source of strength that will bring endurance through any experience. As You know, I'm not one to take things lying down. I'm fighting all the way, screaming for Your help, pounding on the closed door of understanding, hounding You with "whys," making a downright nuisance of myself. You know, God, when life was easy, rolling merrily along, I didn't need You enough to shout. In fact it was kind of easy to forget You. Whispering was sufficient. But now life is tough; I'm stunned by its toughness, *and I need You!* Do You hear me now? I'M SHOUTING!

Whatever else may happen, I *know* You will not forsake us. And, in that knowledge, I am comforted. For only through suffering have You been able to draw so near. Your remoteness in the sugarcoated world of self-sufficiency is as nothing compared to Your nearness in the realistic world of relinquishment.

I feel Daisy's cold nose at my ear. Her bright, drooping eyes and wagging rear end snap my mind back to the tasks at hand and remind me that I, too, have to fight. A renewed sense of courage sweeps over me:

... is your life full of difficulties and temptations? Then be happy, for when the way is rough, your patience has a chance to grow. So let it grow, and don't try to squirm out of your problems. For when your patience is finally in full bloom, then you will be ready for anything, strong in character, full and complete.

James 1:2–4

10

Happy Holidays!

CHRISTMAS IS COMING! The best day of all. Are these days numbered, too? I've got to train my mind to not race ahead into tomorrow and stumble over the significance of today. But now holidays carry more than an air of festivity. They carry an air of finality.

> **December 5**   Didn't feel good enough to go to school today. I'm so tired! Mom took me down to Children's this afternoon. Dr. Hays said I have a good case of the "blahs." I guess I do. I just don't understand myself sometimes. I don't understand how I feel in my mind. Slept until suppertime, then went back to bed. Was depressed. Wonder what Christmas will be like. How can it be the same? How can anything be the same?

Christmas this year just has to be special, in order to break through the hovering clouds of despair and uncertainty. But how can it? I don't even know where all the Christmas decorations are! The living room looks like a storeroom: painting supplies, extra boxes, freshly painted kitchen-cabinet doors and drawer fronts drying on stacks of encyclopedias. There's not even room for a tree! Jim suggests we rent a cabin in the mountains, for the week of Christmas. That's it!

It is a good decision, one that adds the needed element of anticipation to the coming holidays. Those few days are a rest for body and spirit. The decor of the house we rent is even red, white, and blue!

"Well, mom," Kim says when she looks through the window, upon arriving, "we're going to feel right at home!"

We gather wood for the Franklin stove, then spend a cozy evening playing Monopoly and eating popcorn. Relief and thankfulness flood my soul in the warmth of our togetherness. It's a feeling of having run away from overwhelming problems. We're free at last!

Waiting for Jame to make his next move, Kim says, without taking her eyes off the Monopoly board, "Mom, you've got to promise me one thing. You know you always take so many pictures of Jame and me at Christmas, well, you can't this year. Tomorrow's Christmas Eve, and I don't want any pictures of me bald-headed, okay? And I don't want to have to wear that wig all the time. You can take pictures outside, when I've got my cap on. Please, mom, don't forget!"

We're not free, really free. Christmas, 1973, is only a time to rest, to enjoy one another, to grasp anew the real meaning of Christmas, to pause. Thank You, God, Christmas doesn't have to be the same to be special. We shouldn't be the same. For the meaning of Christmas should grow and change within us, as each year passes.

Kim wins the game against overloud, good-natured protests of mismanagement of properties! How she loves to play games!

"Okay, gang, to bed, to bed! Sleds are waxed and ready to roll first thing in the morning. We've got cookies to make, a turkey to bake, a Christmas tree to find—*go, go, go!*"

A brother-sister scuffle breaks out as they race upstairs to their bedrooms. Daisy is in the middle, having a ball. Kim shrieks and giggles, as only a girl can! And Jame shouts and groans like a show-biz wrestler getting pinned!

Jim and I look at each other and exchange thoughts. Surely there's no happier sound than listening to one's kids having a good time with each other.

Christmas Eve Woke up when Jame hollered, "Christmas Eve gift." At least he beat dad saying it! [Whoever says that is supposed to get an extra gift from everyone else in the family.] Mom and I made pancakes for breakfast. Jame and I each had one big as our plate! Dribbled food coloring over them, in the shape of a Christmas tree. Mom and I piddled around while the boys went to find out how the skiing was. When they got back, we all drove to Monarch Ski Area. Jame tried skiing, but I chickened out. It kinda scares me, and I don't want anybody to know it.

On the way back we stopped and looked for a Christmas tree. It started to snow big flakes while we were walking around in the Christmas-tree lot! Neat! It was so pretty! But I got cold and was glad when mom said, "This one says (singing) *'Take me along if you love me!'* " Dad tied it to the trunk of the car. Riding back, I thought we probably looked like a picture on a Christmas card. It was snowing so prettily and we were singing Christmas songs.

After we got to the cabin, we decided to go sledding down the road. Boy, it was a blast! My bottom sure did get cold! Daisy just loves the snow. Her legs are so short she gets in trouble running in it, sometimes!

Came back and ate supper, then mom and I made gingerbread-boy cookies. They turned out pretty good! Sang Christmas carols and made decorations for the tree, out of crepe paper and popcorn. Then we played a new game, and mom read us the Christmas story that she reads every year when we get ready for bed. Threw some carrots out in the snow, for Santa's reindeer—*ha-ha!* Roasted some marshmallows in the fireplace and went to bed. I got mad and upset about my wig, but fell asleep happy. Daisy is sleeping with me. Mom and dad are waiting up for Santa Claus—ho, ho, ho—*ha-ha-ha!*

Christmas Day Got up before anyone else (I think!). Then Jame and I came downstairs, as we always do, excited about seeing what Santa had left in our stockings and under the tree. Dad had a fire going, and mom was pouring orange juice. The blueberry muffins she always makes on Christmas morning smelled so good! That's what woke me up! Dad says one of these days he's going to tell mom there's no such thing as Santa Claus, but he hates to spoil her fun! *Ha-ha!*

We had a good time opening all our presents. I gave Jame some red suspenders to hold his pants up, skiing. I always give dad some handkerchiefs and pipe tobacco. I gave mom an ol' antique WELCOME sign, with clasped hands on it. She loved it, of course. I took a picture of her when she opened it.

After breakfast, we all went sledding, even Daisy! Came back to get warm and played games while mom cooked the turkey. She brought some candles, and I made a chain of construction paper rings to go down the center of the table. Had a real good Christmas dinner! Was stuffed, just like that turkey! Played a few more games, then we had to take the Christmas tree down, 'cause we're going back home tomorrow. Jame and I set it up in a snow drift by the front porch. Put some peanut butter on the branches, for the birds. Went to bed pretty tired, but pretty happy!

Slow down, world. I don't want to get off. I just don't want to miss a thing! Days mean life, and life is suddenly so very precious!

December 31 New Year's Eve! Last day of 1973! Got up and fixed myself some breakfast. Everybody else had already eaten. I was lazy! Watched a little TV, sittin' in my new bean-bag, wrapped up in a blanket. Santa Claus had left Jame and me beanbag-pillow chairs in our garage, while we were gone, Christmas! Felt good to snuggle on a snowy morning. Played on my chromaharp [a special autoharp] granny sent me. It's so pretty! Later I cleaned up my room and worked on my drug report for biology. Dr. Hays gave me some material on drugs, which I can use. Mom and I went to a hobby shop this afternoon and I bought some boards to decoupage some pictures on. It was six degrees below zero when we started back home! I'm glad 1973 is over!

So am I, oh, God, so am I! And yet, I can't shake off this feeling of apprehension. I'm relieved to say good-bye to 1973, but I'm afraid to welcome 1974!

January 1, 1974 NEW YEAR'S DAY! Slept late, since I went to bed *so* late! Ate breakfast while watching all the parades on TV. Read a few chapters in my new Nancy Drew book. We spent a cold, lazy day by the fire. After the football games were over, we all walked over to the Kipharts's house for supper. Finished my book under my electric blanket, when I went to bed.

Leaving the holidays behind means moving back to reality. It was time to go back to the hospital.

January 3 Yesterday was the last day of vacation. Didn't sleep too well, but had to get up, anyway. I didn't have to go to school yet, 'cause I had to go back to the hospital—ugh! After we got there, they just kept taking more blood. I thought they would never quit! I got kind of sick watching it. Sure hope everything's okay.

Kim sits on the edge of the examining table, feet crossed in red, scuffed tennis shoes and white knee socks, pulled up smoothly over her taut, slim legs. Her fist is buried in a tight nest of lap wrinkles. The sleeve on her other arm is rolled up, tight, to the shoulder. Her face is literally drenched in apprehension. I'm standing on one side of the table, reaching for the buried fist. Mary Jo is on the other side of the table, turning Kim's slender arm to the smooth, white underside already marred with grayish blue spots. Hope leaves many scars in its pursuit. We're trying to make jokes about what vein looks the fattest today.

In plunges the needle. Frequently the vein collapses, and another has to be found. Kim cries out in pain. Mary Jo and I continue talking, drawing Kim into the conversation, telling riddles, jokes, *anything* to get a look of relief from that fear-struck, tear-stained face.

The needle releases blood into a vial for testing, and, with a change of vials, becomes a channel through which medication flows back into the veins, to be carried through her system—a fresh supply of battle ammunition, calling in the reserves to active duty.

Glucose solution becomes a highway patrol, Vincristine becomes a paramedic unit, rushing from a feeder street into the traffic flow of a busy interstate network of veins, jammed somewhere along the way with what doesn't belong. Leukemic cells become sluggish wide-load trailers, stalled trucks, speeding cars out of control. Clear out! The flashing red lights of medical science are on the job! Be patient, white blood cells, red blood cells, platelets—help is on the way!

"It's nearly over, Kim," Mary Jo says in a steady voice, her eyes riveted to the tedious focal point of the task at hand. Kim squeezes the buckeye harder, in my hand, and we haltingly begin to sing our favorite little pain ditty, "Oh beautiful, beautiful Texas. . . ."

The crew in oncology loves to tease us about our Texas accents. Of course we pick up the ball and play it to the hilt, so thankful for a source of laughter and lifting of spirits.

Singing this little song helps dull the painful procedures of chemotherapy so many times that we nickname it the "pain ditty." Kim's voice often stalls and chokes with tears before she finishes singing it, but she always finishes. In the days to come, we will sing it together many times.

11

Entering a New Year

WITH A SENSE OF RELIEF and determination, I thumbtack a new calendar to the pantry door: 1974. My warrior spirit races to get ahead of the apprehensive thoughts of what might take place during the turning of each of those twelve pages. Picking up the bottom half of the calendar, I let each page flip slowly back into place: twelve pages of squares, squares with revalued numerals. They seem to become windows of a passenger train through which my fixed stare views the too-swift passing of time. The lines of weeks are as passenger cars, coupled by Sundays. I'm walking through one car at a time. Sometimes it feels as if I'm on a silver streak. The view is a blur. Then, suddenly, I feel the sensation of riding a steam-powered narrow gauge, chugging along steep mountain rails. The view is sharp, at times painfully clear.

As the hours slowly recede, I'm glad it's not possible to see beyond the square window of each day. I'm glad I don't know who or what is a passenger in the car ahead. I'm glad I don't know the final destination. We must be more thankful for the depots of rest along the way; where we get off; wiggle our toes in the green grass of hope; bask in the sunshine of normalcy; and drink at the fountain of faith before once more heeding the call of "all aboard." We must not worry so much about the next station, whether the next sign fixed on the weathered boards of time spells *death*. But God is the engineer. He doesn't need me leaning out the window, giving directions. My trust is the only thing He does need.

January 31   D-DAY—BONE-MARROW AND SPINAL TAP DAY! Went to school, and mom picked me up at 1:00, to go to the hospital. I don't see why I have to go, when I'm feeling good! I get so scared, and it hurts so badly! They gave me a shot this time, and it wasn't too bad, but I was still scared! They don't have a shot for *that!* Slept it off in a bed in the tonsillectomy ward. Dr. Hays let me look at my bone marrow, through the microscope—weird! It was nearly dark when we got home. I didn't know I could feel so tired.

Clinical Data—January 31: "... Spinal tap clear. Remission." Thank You, God! We're still flying! "I am radiant with joy because of your mercy, for you have listened to my troubles and have seen the crisis in my soul" (Psalms 31:7).

February 1   Barely made it through school. My back started bothering me! Could hardly sit up at my desk! Slept, after I got home, until suppertime. After supper I lay down on the couch and played gin with dad, and he beat the tail off me!

Daisy is sleeping in Jame's beanbag chair, next to my bed. Mom doesn't know it!

It's hard to believe I'm okay, when I feel so bad.

February 2   Tried to clean up my room, but started having real bad headaches! It's awful pressure, just pounding inside, like a hammer. Feels better when I'm lying down, but can't get much done that way. When my headache was better, I'd get up and work real fast, then go lie down, when I couldn't stand it any longer. Felt like a jumping jack all day! Took a bath and shampooed my "fuzz" tonight.

February 4 Went to school, but by third hour my headache was so bad I went to see Mrs. Buckley. Had to go home again! Didn't sleep too well. I'm getting tired of this!

February 5 Played it safe and just stayed home today!

February 6 By morning it had snowed five inches! And I was afraid winter had come and gone! I love the snow. Made it all day at school—*whew!* Have a lot of make-up work to do. All day I felt depressed and kind of mad at everyone. I tried to stop, but I couldn't. It's not funny, but sometimes I just can't help how I feel! Maybe something is the matter with my brain.

February 8 At noon, mom picked me up at school, to go back to the hospital. Had a blood test made, and they gave me a shot. Don't have to go back to that hospital for a whole month! *Yea!* I was hungry as a bear all day, probably a reaction to this medicine—ha-ha!

The snow is melting—*pooh!*

February 14 Happy Valentine's Day, 1974! Cupid (?) brought me a midriff blouse. It's darling! Dad didn't much like it though, and Jame kept teasing me about my belly button showing. Mom and I have a hard time with the boys sometimes!

After school I made little Jell-O valentines for our supper and to get extra credit for my home ec. class. Then, after supper, I made our traditional family valentine cake. It was a two-layer, heart-shaped, strawberry cake, and mom hardly helped me at all. If I do say so myself, it tasted dee-licious! We had a good time, as usual, opening our family valentines and reading them to each other.

February 18 George Birthington's Wash Day! It's a holiday today, even though his birthday isn't until Friday. Mom took Brenda and me to the shopping center. Tonight we did our nails and talked. Painted flowers of red polish on each nail—even my toenails! That ought to surprise 'em next time I go to the hospital! Mrs. Fowler, mom's best friend in Houston, taught me to do that. She used to paint daisies on her toenails, every summer! She and mom had a wedding business called Daisy, so naturally everything was daisies! My wedding is going to be the prettiest of all—daisies and daisies every-where!

March 13   HAPPY BIRTHDAY TO ME! Well, Kim, you're a teen-ager now: thirteen! WOW! I wanted an angel-food cake, so, for a change, my birthday cake was in the shape of a *cake!* Mom decorated it in pink and white, with pink rosebuds. It was real good and pretty, especially with thirteen candles! When I woke up this morning, all my dolls and stuffed ani-mals were in a big group on the floor, close to my bed, holding a HAPPY BIRTHDAY KIM sign. Some even had on party hats! Saint Charles looked so cute with that polka-dotted party hat on top of his big head! Crepe-paper streamers were strung all across my room, like a spider web. That "birthday fairy" sure was busy last night—ha, ha!

When I went downstairs, mom had happy-birthday signs everywhere. She had the whole fireplace wall decorated. My big baby picture was hung beside a huge flower-painted num-ber thirteen, with a sign that said "YOU'VE COME A LONG WAY, BABY!" My breakfast dishes were china and sterling, and my milk was in a silver goblet, and I had a cloth napkin! That's usual birthday-person treatment, and everybody else has to eat off of paper plates that day! Mom fixed my cinnamon toast in the shape of a one and a three, and lit a sparkler on top, when she brought my plate. You're pretty special around here on your birthday!

Pam came over, and we had hamburgers for supper. Of course we had the magic-circle hunt for my presents. The best present is usually hidden in the clothes drier or the freezer! It was a real happy day. I can't believe I'm a teenager!

Yes, the days were rolling by with a degree of normalcy. "Mom, what am I going to do? The junior-high department at church is having an overnight retreat at Estes Park, in two weeks. What will I do about my wig, when I go to bed? I can't stand to wear it constantly! But what if somebody wakes up before I do and sees me asleep bald-headed?" Did I say *normalcy?* Well, by the standards we were now measuring the days, yes, that was a prime example of a normal problem. And only this time last year, her biggest concern would have been what to wear.

Though the house is looking brighter and more "us," it closes in on me like a fort. Except for the hospital trips, going to church on Sunday, and shopping errands, I don't want to make the effort to get out. Once inside, I am quite willing to shut the gate. And yet a part of me is screaming to get out. I can't stand to open another paint can! The downstairs is looking good, but the upstairs will just have to wait. If anyone but us wants to go up, I'll tell 'em they're fake stairs, and the thirty-two bedrooms are closed off!

Hmm, and *this* was going to be the year I would begin making the break from "Super Mom," although it is a role I thoroughly enjoy. It has always provided the extra outlet for all my creative energies and imaginative projects. A way to test market my ideas! Now that Jame and Kim are teenagers, I need another outlet, and, with our ever-tight budget, one that is financially rewarding.

But what can I do? I can't get back into the wedding-reception business without a lot of contacts. And it seems impossible without my former partner. Besides, it would require commitment. I can't even commit myself to a dental appointment a week in advance!

A regular job, even part-time, seems out of the question. Besides, I realize that I am the pivot around which my family moves. I need to be home, to be available, because every plan has to be made subject to cancellation. The only certain thing about life is its *un*certainty!

One afternoon, Ruby Korb, a delightful wisp of a lady in her mid-seventies, says to me, "Beth, my neighbor Margaret Zoller just found out her daughter-in-law has leukemia. They are just heartbroken. Please go see Margaret. Only someone who is going through the same thing can really help and understand."

I can understand, God, but can I help? I'm still in a state of emotional shock, myself. Is this part of Your purpose?

I go next door, for I do know that only in giving and helping others do we really help ourselves. I am trembling inside, when I ring the doorbell. What can I say, God? To someone in need, what can a stranger say that will be accepted as friendship? I can only give what I have to give: caring and understanding.

I am about to leave, when the door finally opens. On Mrs. Zoller's face is the reflection of deep hurt and confusion I see in my own mirror so many times. It is the beginning of a special friendship, a sharing relationship that will bolster two families struggling with a common enemy.

I tighten the clamp on reality and busy myself with the belated tasks of a newcomer getting acquainted with her community. Leukemia is in check. It has taken on the guise of normality. Now, so must we.

12

A Tear in the Kite

GOODBYE, WINTER! I can't exactly say it's been a pleasure, but we survived you! I just feel better saying, "Hello, spring!" It's so refreshing to once more witness the constantly changing angle of the sun's rays across the front porch and the stubborn survival of crocus bulbs, pushing through the unworked soil of my flower beds. Spring's alarm is going off. The gnarled limbs of the flowering crab-apple tree are literally bursting with popcorn blossoms of pink.

It is springtime in the Rockies, at last; a whole chorus of God's voice bounces off the foothills. We must lift *our* heads, also. I have only to look westward, to the mountains. The melting snow is rushing into crystal waters, tumbling down the mountain's deep purple crevasses, leaving behind dollops of meringue on each lofty peak. The whole earth is ringing out in explosive color, below crackling, clear blue skies. They ring out with "I live," "I am He," "I AM!" "The earth belongs to God! Everything in all the world is his!" (Psalms 24:1).

The sundial of the seasons has stopped at a very welcome position: a position of promise. Thank You, God. I'm awed at the chance for renewal.

Clinical data—May 2, 1974: ". . . ALL in remission."

May 8 I accompanied the choir at school for the first time. It was kind of spooky; but, with practice, I'll get used to it. During English, I got to feeling so bad I had to go to the clinic and call mom. The lady at the clinic acted as if she thought I was faking it, but I didn't feel like explaining anything to her. She wouldn't understand, anyway. I was pretty depressed, by the time mom came after me; but, after sleeping several hours, I felt better. Tomorrow is Jame's *sixteenth* birthday! Jame started working at Jim Dandy's restaurant today. He's a cook and came home smelling like chicken grease! I wish I could work. I'm going to try to get a baby-sitting job.

May 14 I was so tired, at school, that I could hardly sit up. But I was worried, too. Mom went to the hospital yesterday and had minor surgery this morning. She has a fever and can't come home tomorrow. I miss her so much.

My body just couldn't keep up. I tried to ignore the signs of rebellion for months. After a couple weeks' rest, I am ready to tackle life again.

It is one of those slow days, lined with the blahs. Kim comes home from school, and we are relaxing in the den, when the doorbell rings. As I go to answer it, Kim makes a mad scramble to get her wig on.

"Mrs. Jameson?" says a girl with short, fluffy, thick hair. "Hi, I'm Dana Dittmer. Dr. Hays is my doctor also. I have leukemia, too. I wanted Kim to see my hair. It really does grow back!"

Thank You, God. Another shot in the arm—a nineteen-year-old, Colorado, sun-kissed blond from Denver University, who exudes smiling helpfulness and understanding that can only come from one who's been there.

Although Kim's hair is beginning to grow back, there is not enough for her to go without a wig. Nor does Kim believe there ever will be.

"See, Kim, it really is mine." Dana shakes her head. "Only a few months ago, I had to put up with wash 'n' wear hair, too."

Kim wants to believe so badly. To my surprise, she suddenly lets her wig slide off and asks Dana what she thinks.

"Hey, you've got a five-o'clock shadow! I bet by the time school is out it'll be thick enough to just trim around the edges. Everybody'll think you got a summer haircut."

"I sure hope so!" Kim's voice shimmers with renewed hope. It is so much easier for her to believe Dana than what anyone says at the hospital.

> **June 3** Today was *another* worst day of my life! During lunch, a big bunch of boys at my table decided I was wearing a wig and said they were going to take it off. I grabbed my books and just ran out of the cafeteria. Mrs. Buckley knew who some of the boys were and talked to them. She told me later they said they would stop teasing me and wouldn't really do it, but I don't trust them.
>
> The choir concert was tonight, and I accompanied them on the piano for one song. I did okay, but I was nervous. Some of the girls told me the boys were going to try it again. I'm so scared; I don't know what to do!

No, school does not end on a happy note. It is not the usual, jubilant, "Hooray, school's out!" It is an unusual relief, "Thank the Lord, school's out."

> **June 6** We're leaving for Plainview tomorrow. Can hardly wait!
>
> **June 11** Mom and I are in Brownwood, now, visiting mama and papa. Dad and Jame had to go back to Denver. Of course we have Daisy with us, too. She likes to swim in Lake Brownwood as much as we do!
>
> After we left Plainview, I decided not to wear my wig anymore; it's too hot! Besides, I want to go swimming and all that,

and *I hate that wig!* Anyway, the family said I looked good, and I think I do, too. Looks as if I've got a real short boy's-style haircut, and it's getting thicker every day. Can't wait to go to the lake tomorrow. Hope I can still water ski!

June 13 I wanted to water ski real badly, but, after a couple of times, I got so tired I thought I was going to pass out. But I tried. It was more fun floating around the dock, in a big inner tube, trying to hold Daisy! She thinks she's a seal! Went home and rested.

While mama and papa took a nap, mother let me try on her wedding gown, which was hanging in the back of the closet in our room. Man, oh man, is it ever pretty! It has a hoop skirt and yards of lace and everything. Mom said she was saving it for me and got kind of teary. We talked about weddings and everything and how pretty mine was going to be. Sometimes I get so happy talking and dreaming about what I want to be and what I want to do when I grow up, that I forget to worry about *if* I grow up.

June 20 Back home at last! I am so tired that I can hardly think. Had fun on the trip back, though. I called Pam the first thing. Then Tami and I went over to the swimming pool for a quick swim before they closed. A few kids that I knew from school were there, and they said they liked my new haircut. Boy, that really made me feel good.

Summertime, and the livin' is easy. I take Kim to the hospital for blood tests, and all the results come back good. Roll on, you lazy, crazy days of summer!

July 5 Found me a bridesmaid's dress! I sort of wanted a new bathing suit, but mom said we couldn't afford any extras, with Kathy's wedding coming up. Sometimes I think it's because of me that we don't have a lot of extra money to do things with. I wish I could help pay all those doctor bills!

July 19 Great day—I got my ears pierced, finally! Mom called Dr. Hays to see if it was okay, and it was. So we went to Joslin's and had it done in the jewelry department. Thinking about it maybe hurting was worse than it was. It only hurt a second. Dad doesn't much like it, I don't think. Mom got the downstairs bathroom finished, and it's so cute! She put all sorts of darling knickknacks on the wall. Hope I grow up with her talents and tastes.

July 24 Tami came over this morning, and we practiced "The Entertainer" some more. We're getting real good!

Pam came over to spend the night. We rode our bikes to the Pizza Hut for lunch. Would you believe bubble gum went from one cent to two cents? Talk about inflation! Made cookies tonight and played Monopoly with dad. He beat the tar out of us, but we had fun. After we went to bed, I tried to talk to Pam about God and witness to her, but I get backed up into a corner. Maybe next time.

August 5 Mrs. Winans gave me a whole month off from piano lessons, but I still have to practice! Right before going to sleep, I looked in last year's diary. One year ago today I was having those awful pains before I was diagnosed with leukemia. Wonder what I'll be writing about this time next year.

August 8 At noon tomorrow Gerald Ford will be our new president.

We are not watching the television at noon, August 9, for August 9 is also bone-marrow day. Our thoughts and prayers are pouring into Children's Hospital, not Washington, D.C. Jim and I are enduring another long, anxious wait.

Clinical data—August 9, 1974: "Patient clinically well, in for routine pulse phase. Lymphocytes occupy 6% of total count, but about half of these appear to be malignant lymphoblasts."

The kite of remission has developed a tear, just enough to bring about the possibility of its coming down. Although Dr.

Hays still considers Kim in remission, she is quite concerned that the leukemia is smoldering again.

My spirit is scalded. Fear rises once more, scraping my insides raw with icy fingers of doubt. Battalions of methotrexate pour into Kim's veins, trying to repair the tear. The kite is faltering, flying crazily, its tail of hope flopping uncertainly. Dear God, help us to hang on! Peace of mind is so transitory.

Another long ride back home in thought-heavy silence broken occasionally by feeble attempts at light conversation. Kim is lying down in the front seat, her head at the edge of my lap, under the steering wheel, exhausted from the whole painful ordeal. How am I going to manage my emotions this time? Mama and papa are at our house, visiting, before we all go to Aspen for a family wedding. I just can't let my anxiety spoil the happy mood that's been set by the wedding plans and family reunion. Once again I'm struggling to hide aching fears behind a curtain of laughter and gaiety.

Mama and papa are sitting in the porch swing, reading the evening paper, when I pull into our driveway. "Well," papa says, walking over to the sidewalk, "and how was the doctor, Kimberlie Beth?"

"Oh, she was fine," Kim answers weakly, getting out of the car, "It's *me* that's not so hot." Papa chuckles and gives her a kiss. "Mom, I'm going on up to my room, okay? I don't want any supper. Will y'all excuse me? It's been a long day."

She covers up the traumatic effects of the afternoon very well. So must I. Jim arrives home from work. Jame calls from the door, "Mom, we need to eat pretty soon. I have to work tonight." All the normal sounds of a family gathering together again, in the evening, are heard. But my thoughts are in the stillness of an upstairs bedroom with the door closed.

At the supper table, I steer the conversation away from our day's experiences, assuring my parents that everything's fine, that Kim just needs to rest a day or so, that the tests and treatments are an ordeal we have become accustomed to.

Boy, that's a good cover-up line, Beth. Stay calm. Finish cleaning up the kitchen. It will be time to go to bed pretty soon. There you'll have the solitude you need, to let go.

As we put away the leftovers and load the dishwasher, I can hardly keep up with mama's conversation, because of the one I am carrying on with myself. My head is reeling with nonstop conversation, like a control tower guiding an inexperienced pilot to a safe landing.

But I'm Crashing! I can't blink away any more tears. I cannot continue clearing my throat to keep my voice steady. I return the centerpiece to the table and hang up the cup towel.

"I'm going upstairs to see about Kim, mama. Y'all go ahead and watch the inauguration."

No one sees me open the door to the basement. Closing it softly behind me, I run down the stairs and stumble to a lawn chair. In the cool darkness my body and spirit collapse. "Come, Lord, and show me your mercy, for I am helpless, overwhelmed, in deep distress; my problems go from bad to worse. Oh, save me from them all! See my sorrows; feel my pain; forgive my sins" (Psalms 25:16–18). "To you, O Lord, I pray. Don't fail me, Lord, for I am trusting you. . . . None who have faith in God will ever be disgraced for trusting him. . . . Lead me; teach me. . . . I have no hope except in you" (Psalms 25:1–3, 5).

I don't remember going back upstairs. But the next morning I do remember waking up and knowing that my body has once more survived the clammy sweats of fear. I have been refreshed with the cooling breezes of courage and faith.

August 14 Did my housecleaning chores, then pinned the pattern for my plaid jumper all by myself!

Aunt Martha and Uncle David came about noon, from Charleston, Illinois. Boy, we sure do have a houseful of company! Aunt Martha gave me some beautiful, pearl, pierced earrings.

Went with papa and Uncle David to the swimming pool, but I was so tired. Came back to a huge supper: roast, corn on the cob, baked potatoes—the works!

I've been so tired today and depressed, too, even with all the excitement going on. Man, that really makes me mad. I'll get up to do something, and fifteen minutes later I'll be totally exhausted! I'd just like to know when this medicine is going to start helping me, instead of hurting me!

Kim does improve, during the next few days. Her strength and coloring catch up with the excitement. Our anxieties are buried beneath the gaiety of a family wedding.

"Don't worry," Dr. Hays tells me on the phone. "Just have a good time, have fun, and try to forget as much as possible. All of you need a holiday."

We do. It is a fun time, a beautiful time of all of our family being together.

My heart swells with pride as I watch Kim standing at the altar, beside Kathy, holding her bouquet of lacy spring flowers. I've never seen her lovelier. She looks so tall and grown up. Jim and I clasp hands, stunned at the seemingly sudden emergence of young womanhood in our pretty, poised daughter. *Only God will ever know just how much I love that girl!*

Kim's tanned good looks belie the calmed turmoil of leukemia, asleep in her body. No one would ever suspect—who didn't already know.

August 21   Company is packing and going back home. Uncle David played chess with me this morning and smeared me, of course! Thought he ought to take me out to lunch for that, and he did! Boy, was that nice! Got dressed up and everything! He took me to the Greenhouse Restaurant at the Denver in Southglenn and treated me as if I was a real special date or something. That was so nice. Then he bought me a pair of earrings. He is so nice to me!

After they all left, I decided I'd better start getting physically fit for school, so I jogged around the block. But I was so pooped when I got home, that I don't think that's such a good idea! Seems as if the more I want to do, the less I can! My body and brain just aren't cooperating. Makes me mad. My energy is in my head, instead of my legs!

August 24   Took a shower tonight, and, when I got back to my room and combed my hair, it started falling out! I'm awfully scared. I called mother, and she said it was probably because of all the medicine I've been taking lately, and it would probably stop when they changed my medication. I pray that she's right, 'cause I just don't think I can go through it again. I'm in bed, still shaking 'cause I'm so worried. I can't think of anything else. And school starts next week! What am I going to do? I'll just have to pray and have faith in the Lord.

My heart sinks as I escape to my bedroom and shut the door. Oh, God, no! Please! Is there enough courage in all the world to get us through that experience again? Help us, it just doesn't make sense to make a U-turn when we were making it!

I kneel on the floor beside our bed, my hand reaching out for Jim, already asleep. "Jim?"

"What's the matter, Beth?"

"Jim," my voice drenched in tears, "Kim's hair is coming out again."

"Oh, no."

13

A Token of Friendship

August 25   Woke up all upset about my hair falling out. Finally calmed down enough to get ready for church. I wore the denim outfit I made and my new shoes. I looked great, but felt awful! Took a nap after we got home and worried most of the afternoon. Practicing the piano helped. First thing tomorrow morning I'm going to call Dr. Hays. I'm scared to hear what she might say, but I've just got to know if I'm going to be bald again!

August 26   When I woke up there was a lot of hair all over my pillowcase! Oh, I'm so worried! Mother called Dr. Hays, and she told mother it was because of that shot of Vincristine I had and that my hair should stop falling out pretty soon. I pray that it will! I'm still worried, but am sort of relieved.

August 28   I'm so confused, my hair is supposed to stop falling out, but it's not! I'm almost convinced now I'll have to get another wig, and school's fixing to start. I'm so upset! I don't know what to do!

   Pam went with me to church tonight. I'm glad I have her for a friend!

August 29   My hair is falling out more and more. Mom is taking me to the hospital tomorrow, and we'll find out what's going on, I guess. I practiced and sewed all day today to help take my mind off it. I don't want to go anywhere or talk to anybody. I was real happy about school starting and everything, but now I don't want to go at all.

ONCE MORE I'M EMPTYING clumps of hair from Kim's wastebasket, keeping her comb and brush clean, changing her linens every day, while she's out of her room, gathering up hair off the bathroom floor and around her bed. Oh God, my heart is breaking for my child.

Clinical data—August 30, 1974: "Mild hair loss. Kim is depressed and refuses to be out of house. Had a long talk with Kim and mom. Will hear from them next week."

Mild hair loss quickly becomes moderate. And moderate is becoming severe. We have to go back for another wig. There is no choice.

"I'm not going down again to try on wigs! I'm tired of looking at myself as some sort of freak! My friends have seen me with my own hair short all summer. Don't you think it'll be kind of strange if I show up Tuesday with a whole lot of hair? Hair can get shorter overnight, but it sure doesn't get longer! It's just too much to worry about again. Just get me a tutor."

Sitting at the foot of her bed, my hand rests on the soft mound of Kim's quilt-covered feet. Every piece of my heart is in fervent prayer for my child, for courage and strength to replace her despair.

"Mom, I'm just so tired of it all. It doesn't seem to do any good."

"Kim, baby, please don't give up. You've gone so far. Remember the kite? How it struggles to rise against the wind? That's the only way it will fly, and it *must* fly, to accomplish its purpose."

I hold her in my arms, to steady her wrenching sobs. How much more, God? How much more is required? Is Your plan and purpose worth the struggle? We want to hang in there, God, but it gets so hard. Courage has fled again, dragging hope and confidence with it. Our rain barrel is cracklin' dry again, God. Fill it, please.

I must think of something special for us to do, to take her mind off this fearsome problem, to somehow make her receptive to the idea of getting another wig. It must be bought today! The stores will be closed Monday, Labor Day. She is afraid she will see one of her friends. Please, God, we need a miracle, but fast!

"Bye, mom. See ya, Kim," Jame hollers from downstairs. "I'm going to work now."

From her bedroom window, Kim watches Jame get in the car with Bruce. She says softly, "There he goes, not a care in the world."

It's too much. "I'll be right back, Kim." I rush down the hall, to my bathroom, locking the door behind me, reaching out simultaneously to flush the commode and turn on the sink faucet.

I bury my face in a towel as my soul struggles for peace. I don't know how long I sit there on the floor, my head finally raised and leaning against the shower door, looking up at a piece of clear blue sky through the half-open window. The longer I sit looking up, the more at peace I feel.

Dear God, You probably get pretty tired of my asking for help. But there's not a day that we don't need it! How insufficient we are! Thy sea is so great, and our boat so small! And there's a storm at sea. I'm not asking for a sudden stroke of calmness, a sudden deliverance from these choppy waters, because I see how the buffeting has already strengthened and reinforced, molded and waxed our craft for greater durability. And I'm glad. I'm glad it's not the same rigged craft, moored safely along man-made shorelines, anchored in sand. I accept the fact that our future is obscured, that You are the guiding force on this voyage. I'm just asking for direction.

The name, the idea, come to me as clearly as if I heard it spo-

ken: Art Gore. Take her to see Art Gore. That's it. I get up
quickly to find the brochure of photographic paintings by this
exceptional Colorado photographer-artist.

Kim and I discovered his work only last week. From a distance, I thought his photographs of America's rural past were
paintings. But they were no less the work of a gifted artist.

You must be a very special person, Mr. Gore. Your soul
reaches through the lens of your camera.

I go to Kim's room. "Kim, get up and dress. I've got a surprise
for you! We're going somewhere. I'm not going to tell you where,
but you're going to love it! Now, hurry!"

I don't wait for a response, but, as I go downstairs, I hear her
go into the bathroom. Thank You, God, she's getting dressed.
She's going!

I decide to call ahead and see if the studio is open. Surely it is
on Saturday. But I really want to know if there's a chance to meet
Mr. Gore. That's the impetus we need. What am I going to say?
"We like your pictures, Mr. Gore, and want to meet you"? How
many hundreds of times has he heard that! But he's got to know
how important this meeting is.

The warm voice of the lady who answers makes it easy to in-
troduce myself. I hate to crack the door of my soul to someone
we don't know, but I must ensure this meeting. I tell her that Kim
has a physical problem that is depressing her and affecting her
relationships with others.

"Art is here and would love to meet you and Kim," she responds. I feel better already. Thank You, God, I know this is
going to work!

We head our car toward the picturesque little town of Morri-
son, where Mr. Gore's studio is. The main business street is only
three blocks long, dominated by quaint little shops, beckoning
art, and antique browsers. I park in front of a white, wood-frame
gallery, fronted by a modest sign.

"Mother, this is Art Gore's studio! I thought he lived way off somewhere. Is this the surprise? That's neat!"

"Well, then, let's go in."

I'm breathing another prayer, reaching for the screened door. Kim steps in ahead of me and is suddenly greeted by an outstretched hand.

"Hi, Kim! Hello, Mrs. Jameson."

Kim's face wears a surprised look of sheer joy. I am stunned. How does he know who we are? Of all the people leisurely coming and going through the gallery this Saturday morning, he knows! Thank You, God.

He begins showing us through the gallery, explaining his latest projects, telling us how he became interested in photography. He even shows Kim his very first camera, a little box Kodak. I watch the instantaneous happening of friendship stretch minutes of knowing into years. I soon realize that Art Gore is more than a gifted artist; he is gifted with a feeling for man.

Kim is spellbound. Her eyes begin to sparkle at his undivided attention. He even has her laughing over stories of how he obtained some of the props used in the pictures. Before showing us the darkroom, he picks up a magazine from his desk. After signing the cover, he hands it to Kim.

"Here, Kim. This is the latest issue of *Colorado* magazine."

"Oh, that's one of your pictures on the front," Kim exclaims. "Thank you so much."

"And here's a collection of prints I call *Afterglow*. I've written a verse for each one. You and your mom will enjoy reading it."

I glance at the inked inscription on the inside cover: "To Kim, with lots of love, Art." Kim tightly clutches the magazine and booklet. "I don't know what to say. Thank you so much, Mr. Gore."

"Come on," he says, enjoying our visible pleasure. "Meet the gang out back."

Kim throws me an excited glance as we follow Mr. Gore into a comfortably cluttered workroom. Is this the same Kim I brought here an hour ago? I'm so thankful I can hardly keep back the tears.

After he shows us how the pictures are matted, framed, and stamped with his initial seal of wax, I feel we must not take more of his time.

"Wait just a minute. There's something my new friend Kim has to have."

Kim and I look at each other wonderingly, as he walks away. When he returns, he is carrying a large, framed picture.

"Kim, this is for you—just a token of friendship, and, I hope, the beginning of a long, beautiful friendship."

We're both speechless as he hands Kim a dramatic photograph of a red, dew-kissed rose, fully open. Its long stem is entwined with the stem of a dazzling white rosebud, its head snug against the red's calyx. Against a stark, black-velvet background, the roses are caught in a thin ray of bright sunlight.

My eyes see the eternal promise of everlastingness, bracing a life that, through struggle, has opened and, now, too soon, threatens to shatter. As if the white bud is saying to its crimson counterpart, "I'm here. Your life's stem is meshed with mine. Don't despair, when your dew-kissed petals lose their grip and the time comes for them to fall. Don't despair, for I am here, underneath it all."

Tears flow freely down Kim's cheeks as she turns to hug an emotionally touched Art Gore. She manages a choked thank-you, over his shoulder. "I love you, Mr. Gore."

"And I love you, too, Kim. I sure needed a new friend like you! You're going to come back and see me now, aren't you?"

My heart is bursting at this rare moment of strangers becoming friends, of Kim's spirit mending before my eyes. How does he know the extent of our need in such a moment? Nothing has been said, during our visit, to reveal our problem.

Art Gore is God's answer to my prayer. He magnificently fills the need for a miracle. It is the beginning of a beautiful friendship, an important relationship that will bolster our spirits, more than once.

Kim's fingers curve tightly around the framed picture, held against her knees, as she sits beside me in the car. "Mother, he really cared about me. Can you imagine? Art Gore, *the* Art Gore, really cared about me! I just can't believe it! He is so nice, the most important person I've ever met, and he liked me—*me*, a kid!"

I drive around the corner, smiling through a mist of tears. Art Gore, you'll never know how much I love you for this, for the gift of restoring self-confidence and courage in my child. You breathed life into a defeated spirit.

"Mom, I do care, really. Mr. Gore made me see how important it is to care, how much of life is beautiful! Even though he didn't know me before, I think he knew I had given up about something. So, I want to try again. Let's go on downtown and get another wig, before we go home."

I squeeze her hand and reach for a tissue. We have cried together too many times to be embarrassed now! Thank You, God. Bless you, Art Gore.

The phenomenal success of Art Gore, photographer, was very evident on those gallery walls. But the success of Art Gore, the man, is just as evident on the glowing face of my daughter, Kim.

14

Another Reprieve

September 3   Got up early so I'd have plenty of time to get ready and fix my wig. I was really depressed about it yesterday, trying to get it to look right, but Pam came over and helped me. She gave me a real pretty cross necklace. I love her so much! Mom talked to me last night and tried to make me understand that I can live through this. And, if I keep trying and have a good attitude, it will help other people to have courage when they have problems. If I can have enough faith to do that, school will be a lot better for me. It wasn't too bad today. Nobody noticed my wig, I don't think, except Wendy. Boy, was that a relief! Don't really like my classes or teachers, but maybe I'll like them better, as time progresses. First day is always such a hassle.

September 9   Stayed after school and joined Pep Club. Hope I can do it. I wish I could be a cheerleader some day. Tami is going to help me learn some cheers. I am so sick of being tired all the time! There's so much I want to do!

WE EASE INTO ANOTHER FALL. Days drip off the calendar like honey from a spoon, diluted only by regular trips to Children's Hospital. With another vigorous attack from Vincristine and methotrexate, the disease cools off once more. Going for treatments, having to contend with the drugs' side effects—mouth ulcers, nausea (we never know what to expect)—again become irritating nuisances to Kim. She hates the interruptions in her busy life.

October 11 Went to the hospital and got a shot and had a bunch of blood tests made. *Ugh!* I'm getting so sick of all this. Sometimes I wish I were dead!

October 30 Well, she did it again—mom pulled another blooper! Today was the Halloween party at Children's, which Candlelighters organization puts on for kids at the hospital. Mom was supposed to decorate the refreshment table, and I went to help her. Everybody was told to wear a costume, and since Mom thought the witch would be too scary for the little kids, we decided to dress just alike, as country clowns going to the city. We both wore striped overalls; tuxedo cardboard shirt fronts with big rhinestone buttons; great, big, polka-dotted bow ties; black, felt derby hats; and tennis shoes with patches on the toes. Made up our faces cute, too. Anyway, we loaded up the car and took off. We laughed about how embarrassed we'd be, all dressed up like that, if we had a flat! Wouldn't you know it, mom ran out of gas halfway to town. Thank goodness we were close to a station. I wanted to crawl under the seat, but mom got tickled and started laughing! She said she thought it would be funnier if we just played it cool and acted as if we weren't even dressed weirdly. I thought I would crack up when the attendant came over, and she just told him real calmly to "fill 'er up"! He kept staring at us all the time he was using the gas pump. When he got through, mom handed him the money, in her white gloves, and started the car. He just stood there, grinning. Then she said, "Happy New Year," and took off! We were laughing so hard the tears nearly ruined our makeup! That was so much fun; you never know what to expect with mom!

October 31 BOO! The ol' witch was back, bigger and better than ever!

We roll, as gently as a falling aspen leaf, into a quiet November. The whole earth goes to sleep beneath my feet, snuggling under sheets of topsoil, waiting to disappear under a blanket of snow. It isn't dying, it is sleeping, with the Creator's promise of waking to spring's hallelujah.

> **November 3** When I woke up this morning and looked out my window, I discovered a blanket of snow that covered the whole view. It looked so beautiful on the trees, bushes, fences, and just everything! It makes the whole world look so fresh and clean. Today really turned out neat, and I thank the Lord for it.
>
> **November 5** Today I really felt down. Am worried about having a bone-marrow and spinal tap done on Thursday. Also I stuffed my face most of the day. That makes me mad! I hope it's the medicine, otherwise I'll turn into a big, fat pig! Everything seems to be going wrong. I eat all the time and worry and get mad over anything and everything and really nothing! I'm going to bed before something else happens!

At ten minutes before one, Thursday, Kim and I drive into the hospital parking lot. "Dad is coming just as soon as I call him," I tell Kim. "Don't worry now. Everything is going to be just fine. Here's a little extra courage." I give her a tight hug, and we get out of the car. "O God . . . I am trusting you! I will hide beneath the shadows of your wings until this storm is past" (Psalms 57:1).

Clinical data. "ALL in remission." It's impossible to describe the relief that comes with reprieve. Thank You, God. Leukemia is in check, but the price Kim pays in side effects is high.

> **November 11** Today was probably one of the worst days of my life. I made it to school, but, by third hour, my head was pounding so bad I couldn't stand it! I went to the clinic and stayed there through homeroom and lunch. Felt a little better

after lying down. I was determined not to miss my classes, and barely made it to the end of school. But then there was a Pep Club meeting, and, if I didn't go, I would lose points, so I stayed. Nobody could ever guess just how awful I felt. But I don't want to miss anything! Went to bed exhausted. I'm so glad this day is over with!

Leukemia, you are such a spiteful, implacable enemy! Even when you're asleep, you seem to enjoy the adverse effects of all the drugs Kim has to take in order to fight you. It's a savage game of hide-and-seek you're playing!

Kim gradually regains strength and energy. She is adjusting well to the increased dosages of drugs. Again the calendar begins to fill with preholiday activities. I don't want to miss a thing! This year we will have the most beautiful, most special Thanksgiving and Christmas ever!

Christmas Eve Everyone in the family beat me saying "Christmas Eve gift." Pam spent the night with me last night, and we stayed up pretty late. We made some snickerdoodles, but they didn't turn out too well. Jame ate most of them, but then he'll eat most anything! It started snowing, and I'm so happy! We're going to have a white Christmas after all! Everything looks so pretty! Helped mom do some more baking today and some last-minute shopping.

Tonight we went to Calvary Temple Church for a special observance of the Lord's Supper. It was so meaningful. Then we went downtown to St. John's Cathedral to hear parts of the *Messiah*. It was so beautiful I got goose bumps! That cathedral is huge and so beautiful. When we were walking back to our car, it was snowing, and the lights from the tall, stained-glass windows reflected on the snow, just like a scene on a Christmas card.

After we got home, Jame and I roasted marshmallows, and

mom read the Christmas Story and "The Night Before Christmas." Fixed Santa Claus a snack and threw some carrots out in the front yard! Ha-ha! It's late, and I'm pooped. But I feel so good and safe inside. Wish I could always feel like this: Wish everything could always be this beautiful, and I could always be this happy.

Christmas Day MERRY CHRISTMAS! This morning I beat everybody saying "Christmas Gift!" Jame and I were so anxious to go downstairs! Of course mom made us wait until she had the camera ready and dad had the tree lights all on and the Christmas carols playing on the stereo! There are times when tradition can try one's patience! Wouldn't have it any other way, though! The first thing I saw, of course, was my bike. Yea! It's just like the one I picked out. I love it! It's a green Schwinn racer. Jame got a stero tape deck that he sure does like. It was pretty noisy around here today! Mom really does like the patchwork pillow I made for her. She put it on top of the little milk stool in the hall. We had delicious blueberry muffins for breakfast. Tried out my bike about noon, but it was slightly hard, riding it on the icy street! Had Christmas dinner about five. It was *great*, just like Thanksgiving! We all watched "Scrooge" on TV tonight. This bed sure feels good tonight! It was such a happy day.

Oh, God, is *this* the last Christmas our family will be together? Is that why this day is so beautiful?

> For having brought us this one year more,
> I give thanks for depths of joy not known before,
> Joys that only pain could have wrought,
> Courage that only trials could have brought.
>
> For lessons you've taught, for hope to endure,
> For strength when there was none, our faith to secure.
> What lies ahead? Only You can know the days afar,

and see, through the darkness, the reason.
Help us, keep us looking up, following in the
    light we *can* see, from the star of this blessed
    season.

The fun-packed holidays burst and dwindle away after New Year's Eve. Nineteen seventy-four was no more.

15

The Battered Kite of Hope

I TACK MY NEW CALENDAR to the pantry door with renewed determination. January, 1975: a new year—Kim is going to make it; she has to! She will dumbfound them all: the doctors, nurses, lab technicians, researchers—she will beat this lawless invasion of leukemic cells.

> **January 1** HAPPY NEW YEAR! Made it through another one! I hope what I write in here isn't all that depressing, but I know a lot of it will be, because, if I write my thoughts down, I can get them out of my head and be a happier person, at least for a while. This sounds awful, but sometimes I want people to feel sorry for me. (If somebody ever reads this, well, please try not to.) But is it wrong? I mean, *all* this I'm going through, I want a little sympathy. I sort of need it. But not too much! I'm strong and able and can fight this queer disease until I'm just as well as anybody else! *And that's what I'm going to do!*

Jim is driving me to Swedish Hospital. The gray clouds of this crisp January day are swirling with threatening weather changes. So is my soul. Depression seeps in, like a summer rain, through my crumbling walls of courage. My protective roof of cheer is leaking. I know it's ridiculous, but, in the forced reality of living with the awful possibility of losing a child to cancer, it's hard for a mother to write *finis* to her childbearing years. What if something does happen to Kim? What if she doesn't make it?

Jame is a senior in high school. He'll be leaving home soon. Oh, God, what will I do? My whole life is geared around the family, the role of mother. Though it may seem impractical, thirty-nine isn't really too old, is it, to have another child? Can anyone quite understand how I feel? I'm also afraid. More and more, I feel our presence in a tornadic path from which there's no escape. "O God, listen to me! Hear my prayer! For wherever I am, though far away at the ends of the earth, I will cry to you for help. When my heart is faint and overwhelmed, lead me to the mighty, towering Rock of safety. For you are my refuge . . ." (Psalms 61:1–3).

Flowers and cards arrive to lighten the physical struggle of the next few days. It's Thursday evening, and I'm looking forward to Jim bringing Jame and Kim to visit. Kim did not look well last night. When she gave me the get-well card she had made and leaned over to kiss me, I sensed that something was not right.

My fears become real when the door to my hospital room opens and Jame and my sister Martha come in without Kim.

"Now don't worry," Martha says quickly, "Kim is running a fever, but I've talked to Dr. Hays, and she has already started her on some medicine."

My eyes close in apprehension. Overwhelming weakness dissipates my spirit. I've never known such a feeling of helplessness. Lord God, help us both.

Kim doesn't come the next day either. Jame comes in my room about noon. "Mom, dad and Aunt Martha had to take Kim down to Children's this morning. Her fever got up to one hundred and four. Dr. Hays says it's pneumonia. I know what this does to you, but please don't worry. They're taking good care of her, and it won't help if you get worse. So buck up now, and have faith. We need you, mom."

It's useless to fight the tears; but through them I see a strength in the face of my seventeen-year-old, which I haven't seen before. His faltering efforts to console and cheer loosen the vise around my aching heart.

When Jim brings me home from the hospital, it's Kim opening the back door. She has my pillow and a blanket spread out on the divan. I don't need to be coaxed to lie down. I watch quietly as she helps Jim build a fire in the fireplace and place the flowers we had brought home around the den. We have been through so much together that we have become quite a team. Apart, our courage seems to falter.

The next few days are tedious. I cannot seem to rest well, nor do I have the strength to resume any household duties. What's the matter with you, body? It's time you were mending, shaping up, getting back to work! I have the sickening feeling I am getting worse, instead of better.

Dr. Hays wants to see Kim on Friday. I realize I will not be able to go with her. Jim comes home from work to take her. After they leave, the aloneness, stillness, and quietness of the house close in around me. The dust on my dresser across the room looks an inch thick. The dirty clothes hamper is bulging. The carpet needs vacuuming. And here I am, in bed, just barely able to take care of myself! That old enemy, self-pity, takes over once more as my concern over trivia looms out of proportion.

The phone rings. I reach for it quickly, hoping it's Dr. Hays. But it's a well-meaning friend, wanting to pray and read a passage of Scripture to me, over the phone. Oh, God, I don't need talk! I need prayers that walk!

I hear the back door open and someone come in. "Hi, I know you need your rest, so I'm not going to stay," a voice calls up the stairs. "Thought you might need the bathrooms cleaned. There's a roast on the stove for supper. Call if you need anything. 'Bye."

"Phyllis, thank you so much." Phyllis Kiphart, my neighbor

and friend, can never know the extent of my appreciation. Thank You, God, for prayers that walk.

The phone rings again. "Beth, this is Taru. Kim is doing much better, and I'm not worried about the pneumonia anymore. But I want to do a bone-marrow on her tomorrow and see just what the situation is."

My relief, brought by hearing the first sentence, is quickly absorbed with apprehension, brought by the second. Don't worry, everybody says, "Don't worry." God, how can I help it?

By midafternoon I am running a fever. Jim calls my doctor. "You'd better get her back to the hospital. I'll call ahead and have a room ready."

"Kim, I'm sorry, babe, but I'll get better faster this way and will be home real soon, fit as a fiddle."

But "soon" is to stretch into ten long days. About noon the next day, a nurse hands me the phone. My fingers are icy with fear.

"Beth, I hate to call you at the hospital, but Kim is in a relapse."

My grip on the receiver goes limp. I can hear no more. My whole body tumbles into a vortex of disappointment, despair.

> **February 12**   The bone-marrow today said I was in a relapse. I'm getting a new drug now, called adriamycin. I don't know much about it, except I have to have it. Dr. Hays said they needed a change, because the old drug wasn't working as well. God, I'm so scared.

Oh, my God, here, here's the ball of string, here's our battered kite of hope. Forgive me, but I just do not understand life. Days are just so many hours of complexity, ambivalence, confusion, and uncertainty. Nights are just so many hours of restless sleep, staring at the ceiling, listening to the beat of an aching heart. I'm tired, God, so tired. I'm floating free. Nothing makes sense any-more.

The only direct statement of Jesus which is simple enough for me to comprehend when my heart is breaking or when I'm discouraged or scared is: "Follow me." I can-not understand life because life is not understandable, but I can grasp: "Follow me."

EUGENIA PRICE

Steady me with Your promises, God, that I may believe and be strengthened by them once more. You are no longer a noun, God, in the vocabulary of my life. You are a verb.

16

The Taste of Defeat

COME ON, MARCH, blow! Usher in those seesaw days of springtime in the Rockies—days of snow flurries that frustrate the timid crocuses, taking turns with bright sunshiny days that startle the sleepy trees. We need you, spring! We need to be part of your magic circle of emergence, your stubborn insistence on being.

Though my heart is burdened, my body strengthens rapidly, and is once more ready to fulfill the waiting tasks and responsibilities. I am asked, "Aren't you glad all that's behind you now? Aren't you just feeling great?" How I wish I could stretch my arms; cling to the edge of a fluffy, white cloud; and swing in sheer exuberance, shouting, "Yes, I feel *great!*"

But feelings of body and spirit walk hand in hand. One doesn't leap ahead of the other. Outside I wear the tranquil mask of "all's well." Inside, I am a general getting into uniform, studying battle plans to meet the demands leukemia imposes on the lives of my whole family.

Kim's involved in school, wearing the facade of a carefree typical teenager and handling the increased dosages of chemotherapy well. But the whole family has trouble coping with the complex, dual problem of controlling its own fears and anxieties, while simultaneously supporting and encouraging Kim.

Just the normal process of getting ready for school is an exhausting routine for her. Pain in her back and legs is becoming more severe. But she never once considers missing school, because of the make-up work. She says it is hard enough to keep up with everything as it is. I cannot challenge such a determined display of inner strength. But it hurts to watch her struggle. As Jame remarks, "It's like a long soap opera with no commercials."

In our own way, each of us is caught in the cruel trap of non-being, as if our lives will never be free from leukemia. Kim is not going to die from it, but neither will she ever be cured!

Leukemia has become the elusive castle ghost, an unwelcome entity in our home. Invisible, teasing, insidious, subtle, demanding—forcing awareness of its unrelenting presence, it seems hell-bent on evicting us all.

Anxiety releases untapped energies as I look at the calendar and count eight more days until Kim's birthday. Planning the first family celebration of the new year covers well the struggle and hurts of daily living under the cloud of leukemic relapse.

"Mrs. Jameson? Hi, this is Pam. I'm calling now because Kim is staying after school for a Pep Club meeting. We want to have a surprise birthday slumber party for her at Melissa's house, Friday night. I want to make sure it's okay with you."

That is so like Pam, and it's just what Kim needs. It *is* a fun weekend, a very happy birthday, from the girls' party to the magic circle and birthday spanking. As Jim holds Kim, giggling and screaming, in his lap, never is that extra pat applied with more seriousness. Never have so many wishes gone with that "one to grow on."

Dear Debbie,

Last night some friends at school gave me a surprise birthday slumber party. Took lots of pictures. I'll have to send you some. It was at Melissa Robinson's house. I sort of had a feeling something was up, but was still surprised. We had a spaghetti supper with French bread and salad—*yum!* Then we "monkey walked" around the neighborhood. Wanted to TP Joe's house, but they didn't have any trees or shrubs, and their porch light was on! Came back and had birthday cake and then had ice cube fights—ha-ha! Played Mr. Twister. Generally we laughed and talked—which is what we do best! Only slept about four hours. This morning, when we got up, it was snowing so beautifully—great big flakes.

So, we decided to make a snowman. That was fun! But the sun is out now, and it's warm. Our snowman is probably just a puddle! Had yummy strawberry pancakes for breakfast. Then we all squeezed into Mrs. Robinson's Toyota, and she drove everybody home. Yep, it was a real fun birthday.

I'm glad it was, too, 'cause I've been feeling lousy lately. Have to have a bone-marrow next week. I dread it already.

> Luv ya,
> KIM

I find myself actually looking forward to Kim's coming bone-marrow aspiration. The results have always brought relief from this strained period of relapse.

"Beth," Jim calls from the office, Monday. "I have an appointment Thursday afternoon and tickets to the hockey game. I really need to take some customers. What do you think? I know Kim's bone-marrow is that afternoon. Can you manage at the hospital without me, then meet us in town, for dinner and the game?"

It sounds like a good plan, I tell Jim, a chance to celebrate a new period of remission.

Thursday afternoon, as I sit alone in the oncology waiting room, the apprehension I think is gone comes back and hits me like a truck. I left Kim in the examining room, a few minutes ago, after pressing the shiny buckeye in her hand and brushing at a runaway tear on her anxious face. It will never be easy, will it, God? A bone-marrow will always be hell.

My thoughts are drowning in my cup of cold coffee. Suddenly, over the droning voices on television, I hear Kim scream again and again. The cup drops from my hands. The spilled coffee on my slacks forces me out of the chair and away from the awful reality of what Kim is going through.

No one is in the rest room. My hands grasp the edge of the sink, and my head rests on the ledge under the mirror. Oh, my God, I don't know myself anymore. I don't even recognize the anxiety-riddled face in this mirror. Right now, I feel as if I don't even know You! Why, why does my child have to suffer so? You must know all the answers, for You can see the whole. But I can't! I love Kim so deeply. She is so much a part of me that her pain is also mine.

So, God, since love stands in the way of any acceptable and understandable explanation, give us grace to endure, courage to withstand, and strength in spirit. We are on a path that cannot be walked alone.

An hour passes. I should get back. I'm certainly ready to see Dr. Hays's smiling face and feel the relief of "It's over, and all's well."

As I return to the waiting area, Dr. Hays steps around the corner from the clinic. She is not smiling.

"Beth, why don't you go on into the conference room. I'll be right with you."

Oh, God, no, not the conference room! Every other time we've had to go into the conference room, it has meant bad news. A sickening wave of dread sweeps over me.

Once more I step out of the procession of life. Fear strikes with the severity of instant panic. Words again trigger a volcanic emotional eruption as I lower my head to absorb their crushing impact. The sound of compassionate voices fades into thunderous explosions of terror. I am only aware of my world turning black and pelting my body with dust, choking fragments of hope. Time dissolves into a meaningless void as I grasp the edge of the long conference table and sit. Taru comes in with Mary Jo and closes the door. She sits beside me and rests her hand on my arm.

"Beth, I'm sorry. The increased dosages have not worked. Kim is still in relapse. Her hemoglobin and white blood count are still dropping. . . ." The words fade with the terror ripping through my soul.

"Beth. Beth, Kim needs you."

The spires of my spirit were not very high, anyway, God, and there they go again. But they must be raised, for Kim's sake! Here, God, over here! I'm like a wind chime suddenly blown to the ground by a gust of wind, lying here in a tangled pile of prisms. Help me up! There is still music in me, a song to sing, life! My soul must not remain dwarfed in fear, at this crucial opportunity for growth!

Kim is sitting on the edge of the examining table, slowly putting on her ski jacket, as I walk into the room. Her face is flushed and stained with tears. She reaches out for me and clings to my neck as I hold her close. I whisper to her softly, with a smile. "Hi, babe. Let's go home."

Another unseeing drive toward Littleton—Kim is exhausted and tries to sleep with her head on my lap, under the steering wheel. I'm going through the mechanics of driving, but I really don't feel aware of what I'm doing. How many times we've driven this route, under the weight of anxiety! It's a miracle we've not had an accident.

When we get home, Kim lies on the divan in the den, and I call Jim. We'll have to cancel the evening's plans. I couldn't possibly play the charming-hostess role for strangers. I don't want to see or talk to anyone.

Jim insists he cannot cancel his plans. "I've already talked to Dr. Hays," he says, "we'll discuss everything when we get home. Please, honey. It will be good for you, under the circumstances. I know you can do it."

Jame agrees with his dad, and volunteers to take care of supper for Kim and himself. If Kim has any problems, he is to call Mary Jo or Dr. Hays.

Reluctantly I change clothes, furious at being trapped into an unavoidable social commitment.

God, help me, please. Help me to control my emotions. Help me not to suddenly burst into tears in the midst of light conversation. Help me to concentrate on the game, on the people we're with, on what we're doing and talking about. Help me to think straight, to be able to carry on an intelligent conversation, to calmly field those inevitable questions: "And do you have children?" "How old are they?" "What are their interests?" Help me not to blow it in front of strangers who couldn't possibly understand!

Gradually I switch gears into another me, as if a shield of pretense snaps into place. I'm ready, I hope.

We make it through dinner okay. My concentration is working well, as long as my eyes do not meet Jim's. But I run into trouble at the game. I thought hockey was supposed to be fast, furious, and exciting! Tonight's game drags. My head is in steady rhythmical motions of no, as I watch the players skate rapidly from one goal to the other. Help, I'm losing my concentration! The thousands of people in that arena seem to be shouting "No!" along with the silent screams of my heart. What am I doing here, watching a stupid hockey game, when my child is dying! Oh, my God!

Jim feels me stiffen and reaches for my hand. He pretends to pick something up from underneath his seat. "Hang on, honey. It will be over soon," he whispers.

I take a sip of Coke and force myself to choke in order to excuse the tears spilling down my cheeks. At last the game is over. We say our it's-been-such-a-fun-evening-we-must-do-it-again good-byes in the parking lot.

Since we have both cars, Jim plans to follow me home. But my tears roll out of control. "Jim, I can't drive. I can't get control of myself, I can't."

"You can! I know you can! It's one o'clock in the morning, and we've got to get home. Let's go!"

He gets in his car and pulls up behind me. He's right. I can't give in now; I turn the key in the ignition. Traffic is light. My eyes are damming up a flood of tears. God, help me!

Having to stop for a red light breaks the dam. I can't control the racking sobs. Tears block my vision. When the light turns green I can't move. I have no sense of thinking or feeling, only the stabbing sensation of intense grief.

The sound of Jim's horn snaps me back. He pulls up beside me, gets out of his car, and shouts through the closed window, "Beth, Beth! You *can* make it! Now, let's go!" There is still a spark of "I ain't down yet" buried beneath this heavy load of anxiety, as somehow we make it home. "When the fight begins within himself, a man's worth something" (Robert Browning). "Defeat may serve as well as victory, To shake the soul and let the glory out . . ." (Edwin Markham).

17

The Struggle, Not the Prize

APRIL FOOL'S DAY, 1975—hey, it's the day for fun, jokes, games. Somehow the silly pranks played on each other just don't have the usual punch. The tension of leukemic relapse is stifling our atmosphere. More and more I realize how true it is that cancer may physically strike only one member of the family, but the whole family bears its devastating consequences.

Kim is very depressed over her hair coming out again. The pain in her back is becoming more chronic and severe. She cannot sit comfortably for very long at a time, and she has difficulty walking. Sometimes she looks to me like a little old lady—the slow, faltering steps on the stairway, struggling to keep going. My heart breaks to watch her.

> **April 1** I am so sick of shedding! No one knows what it's like, waking up with your sheets, blankets, pillow, and pajamas full of your own hair! Mom talks about how much trouble it is picking dog hair off the carpet on the stairs; well, if she had to pick about one hundred hairs of her own off her pillow and pajamas *every* morning, she'd have a completely different attitude. That didn't sound very nice, but I'm trying to get it off my mind, and I guess my way of doing it is blaming it on someone else. God, I'm sorry.

Just when my sense of humor is wrung dry, the staff in oncology picks up the ball. When we walk into the clinic, the whole crew is wearing Mickey Mouse T-shirts! The shocked look on our faces triggers laughter that I thought was surely impossible to produce this day. Thank You, God! Kim is delighted at their antics. I don't know what a stranger would think, but under this three-ring-circus atmosphere runs the most efficient, compassionate team of medical personnel, unequaled in their field. The genuine friendship offered patient and family produces confidence and trust.

Laughter and tears are surely close relatives, for laughter is a wonderful solvent, when the grit of despair gets into the cogs of life.

Clinical data—April 1, 1975: "Patient with ALL in relapse after three weeks chemotherapy. Back pain and depressed over loss of hair. Begin L-Asparaginase and return in one week."

"Beth," Dr. Hays hands me some papers, "we need to make a change in Kim's medication. I'm going to start her on a drug called L-Asparaginase. I want you to read about it, and then we'll need your signature on this consent form. Be sure to ask me anything you don't understand. Why don't you step into my office to read? I'll be explaining the procedure to Kim."

Mixed emotions sweep over me again as I slowly sit down to read: disappointment over the drugs that have been used losing their effectiveness, yet hope and relief that another drug is available—fresh troops, new ammunition.

L-Asparaginase has drastic side effects, including usually temporary abnormalities in kidney and liver function, and in blood clotting. In treating sixty-four children with this drug alone, over half achieved significant reduction in leukemia. The potential benefits are the achievement of a long, disease-free remission. This contrasts with the progressive course of leukemia, which ultimately leads to death, if the disease is unchecked.

God, hope is so well camouflaged, concealed in the maybes and maybe nots of medical jargon—from the possibility of a reaction causing death, to the possibility of a long disease-free remission. The responsibility of my signature on that line is so great it's inconceivable. But so is the desire for my child to live. As long as there is a shred of hope, I'll sign—a signature of faith, no guarantees.

Kim tolerates the first dose well, to the relief of us all. Oh, the nausea, fatigue, and stomach pains follow, but Kim forces herself back into the mainstream of school activities.

I discover the truth of G. K. Chesterton's words: "Courage is almost a contradiction in terms. It means a strong desire to live, taking the form of a readiness to die."

Kim lives the reality of Robert Frost's dictum: "Courage is the human virtue that counts most—courage to act on limited knowledge and insufficient evidence. That's all any of us have."

There are no yesterday leftovers of courage.

> **April 20**   I can't explain it, but today I felt the disease. It moved from my chest to my back. It's such a weird feeling to know that is what is causing all the pain I'm going through. I'd give almost anything to be well again!
>
> I just heard this on the radio: "Always give your friends the best, and you'll always have the best of friends." I've got to remember that.

I glance out the kitchen window. There's the school bus, right on time. We'll have to hurry to make our appointment at Children's. Kim needs L-Asparaginase and a blood transfusion today. Wouldn't you know it, just when she's getting over the drug's side effects, it's time to go back for another dose.

"Hi, mom!" The front door slams. I hear the sound of books dropping to the floor. That going-under feeling I had disappears as I catch the lilt in her voice. "Mom, I really had a good day. Can you believe that? I don't even mind going to the hospital!"

"Well, podner, let's head out!"

I reach for my purse, and Kim reaches for the box of vanilla wafers, as we head for the door. She lies on the backseat to rest, but that doesn't stop her chattering. God, thank You for this calming breeze in the midst of our storm!

"Hey, guess what? See this paper? It's a sponsor sheet for the Inter-Faith Task Force twenty-five-mile walk. And guess who signed up to walk it? *Me!*"

I hit the brakes. "You're going to do *what?*"

"Hey, take it easy. All I said was I was going to go on the twenty-five-mile walk for the Inter-Faith Task Force. It's like this: You get as many people as you can to sign up as your sponsors, and they pledge to give so much money per mile that you walk. That's how they raise money, every year, so they can do things for old people and people that need stuff. A bunch of my friends at school were signing up, so I did, too. Great idea, huh? Pam and Keely and I are going together. I'm going to sign up some sponsors at the hospital. Won't they be surprised when they realize it's *me* they're sponsoring for a twenty-five-mile walk? You can be my first sponsor!"

I am speechless. My heart is bursting with pride and admiration. I sign eagerly, although my mind boggles at the impossibility of her accomplishing such a task.

Kim requires two units of blood, plus the L-Asparaginase infusion. It is a long afternoon. Yet the pencil and sponsor sheet never leave her side, in that bed. Her right arm and hand are taped immobile, to a board, for the infusions, but her left hand is ready to grab anyone who comes into her room and sign them up. She has a goal. it is important that she reach it. And not one of the doctors and nurses who signs even hints, "You've got to be kidding."

> Life's battles don't always go
> to the stronger or faster man:
> But soon or late, the man who wins
> is the one who thinks he can.
> "The Victor"
> C. W. LONGENECKER

Sunday morning I deposit three bursting-with-energy teenagers at Littleton High School. It is a crystal-clear, typical Colorado morning. Several hundred teenagers are already in the street when we arrive. The air crackles with picnic anticipation. I give Kim a handful of dimes, to call me at the five-mile rest stops, my only display of anxiousness.

I park the car on a side street, to watch the walkers pass by. What a thrilling sight to see them coming, en masse, from a distance—hundreds of kids of all ages, literally filling the street, curb to curb, united toward the goal of giving to the community.

My mind clicks back to the image of yesterday's Kim, lying in a hospital bed all afternoon, tubes and IV needles, leading to overhanging bottles slowly dripping life into her veins. Today's Kim is one of the crowd, lost in a sea of happy, healthy, tanned bodies on their way to walk twenty-five miles for the benefit of someone else's needs. What a contrast. I rest my forehead on the steering wheel and breathe a prayer of thankfulness. Go, baby, *go!*

There is no reason to worry. As soon as I spot those three in the crowd, I know Kim will make it. They are pushing a young man in a wheelchair. Truly, ". . . the virtue lies in the struggle, not the prize" (R. M. Milnes).

It is a teeth-clattering Kim I pick up at Heritage High School, later that afternoon, in the blinding midst of an early spring blizzard.

"I made it, mom," she manages as I wrap her in a blanket and start for home.

As we pull into our garage, I hear her muffled voice from the blanket, "Mom, I never knew being so tired on the outside could make you feel so good on the inside."

She misses the next two days of school.

18

Return to Remission

CLINICAL DATA—MAY 1, 1975: "Patient with ALL in relapse after three weeks chemotherapy. ALL considered in remission."

There goes our kite again. Though it's not soaring as high as usual, at least it's off the ground. I'm just not feeling the delirious joy that news of remission has brought in the past. The true meaning of that word has finally impacted: a temporary halt of leukemic progression. And *temporary* does not mean "permanent." This extraordinarily complex disease only appears to be permanently halted, just as Kim only appears to look and feel well. My thankfulness is not diminished at hearing the news of remission, but faith in a permanent cure is crumbling.

May 11 Today was a real good day. We got up early and drove to the mountains, for a family picnic to celebrate Mother's Day. It was so beautiful! And fried chicken never tasted so good! Had so much fun exploring the streams and picking up rocks. We even played baseball. Put Daisy in center field and called her Snoopy, but she's not much of a ball player. Kept wanting to play in the water!

Made Mom two cards, 'cause I couldn't decide which one to give her. On the outside of one, I drew clouds and a rainbow and wrote, "God can't be everywhere . . .," and, on the inside,

"... so He invented mothers like YOU! Luv ya always, Kim."
And for the other card, I drew a picture of daisies (naturally!)
and wrote, "Thanks for happening to me! Happy Mother's
Day, Lots 'n' lots of love, Kim." By the way she acted, I knew
she liked 'em a whole lot. I don't know how I'd get along
without mom. She always says just the right words to make
me feel better inside. I love her so much!

I tuck away the memories of Mother's Day, in my heart—a
day of happiness, joy, family togetherness, of just being close to
each other. It even takes away the sting of my having turned the
big 4-0 on my birthday, a few weeks ago. It is to be one of the last
just-fun days our family will ever spend all together.

May 31 Well, here I am again, stuck in the hospital! IVs in
my arm the whole time. Can't even go to the bathroom without somebody having to wheel that dripping-bottle contrap-
tion around with me! Oh, well, I guess I don't mind all that
much, 'cause I was feeling so rotten when I got here and am
feeling a little better now. I'm just mad, 'cause I'm missing the
last few days of school. Glad it's over, though. Sometimes I
wonder if I'd be a lot different now if I hadn't gotten leukemia.
I think I'd probably have a lot more friends, 'cause I wouldn't
be the oddball I am now. I'd also be a lot prettier. My hair
would be so long and pretty. *Why?* It's not fair! If God would
just let me see what His plan is, then I would have something
to push toward and look forward to. Oh, help!

The door to Heaven is wide open to all who will enter,
but the windows are closed—the drapes tightly pulled.
There's no explanation of whys, no understandable clear
answer, no sneak preview of "one day you'll understand."

"Markings"
DAG HAMMARSKJÖLD

June 2 If I have to go through so much pain to stay alive, I'd much rather be dead and in heaven with God.

God, I'm asking that unanswerable, bleak question again: "Why?" But is it so wrong? In a sense I feel relieved to ask, because my pride is shattered, and hope feels betrayed. One's life patterns can crumble so suddenly.

No explanation to suffering can satisfy the heart. But satisfaction does come from talking to You about it. And I guess I don't really need to know *why* near as much as I need to know *how:* How am I going to have the strength this situation demands? How is Kim? How do we become "more than conquerors"?

Turn to Him for something better than explanations. Turn to Him for that ultimate thing, strength to live life out gallantly. He didn't say, "Come unto me and we'll sit and ponder life's puzzles." He said, "Come unto me, all ye that labor and are heavy laden, and I will give you rest."

"The Salty Tang"
FREDERICK B. SPEAKMAN

Kim swings into a happy summer, though teetering on the edges of a cold, a virus infection, a fever, or a sore throat. But each time comes back the happy report that her leukemia is still in remission. None of these ailments has awakened the sleeping giant. Thank You, God, thank You!

19

Do Not Be Anxious

July 31 I got up all worried about going to the hospital. Tried to take my mind off it by sewing, but that didn't do much good. I'm trying to make a dress with a pinafore. The material is navy with white pin dots and red strawberries. I think it's going to be real cute—I hope!

I got the bone-marrow and spinal tap done, except it took 'em twice on the spinal tap, which wasn't very much fun! Came home and rested. Glad that's over for a while. I hope. I think I'm doing okay.

CLINICAL DATA—JULY 31, 1975: "Clinically ALL in remission. Comment: The focal increase in immature lymphocytes is disturbing, but the overall cellularity is in keeping with a remission bone marrow."

Thankfulness skips over my soul like a stone skimming the mirrored surface of a pond. I have finally learned that *remission* does not mean the giant is dead. Therefore, a reaction of ecstasy is replaced by one of quiet relief.

It is clear that Taru is also relieved, as she talks to Jim and me about the bone-marrow results. But she seems anxious to get on to something else.

"It's a procedure that will require your written permission to be used on Kim."

My heart signals red alert to my brain.

"While Kim is in a remission, we feel it is the right time to try something new—immunotherapy through the use of BCG, a live tuberculin organism."

The oncology center is beginning a program of immuno-therapy, starting with leukemia. The National Cancer Institute is supplying the BCG, which is a very potent stimulant to the immunosuppressive system. Generally it revs up the entire system. Preliminary work has already been done in Houston at M. D. Anderson Hospital and at the Trudeau Institute in Canada. Kim would be the first leukemia patient in the Denver area to receive the BCG treatment.

"There's a very good chance that BCG will prolong Kim's remission," Dr. Hays finishes. "It's worth taking that chance."

So BCG is actually another dose of hope, another gentle breeze to keep our kite in the air. I reach for the paper, with a steady hand, eager to know more about our new "partner."

Even though hair loss again painfully glares at us from the list of side effects, Jim and I cannot refuse to allow any treatment of promise to go untried in our daughter. We sign.

> **August 7** After breakfast I got ready to go to the hospital. At least I don't have to worry about having to have a bone-marrow or spinal tap this week. My blood count was up to 1100, which is so-so. They told me they are going to use some new method of treatment called BCG. And I'm the first one to get it in Denver. How about that? But that scares me. What if something goes wrong?

"Will all your worries add a single moment to your life? . . . So don't be anxious about tomorrow. God will take care of your tomorrow too. Live one day at a time" (Matthew 6:27, 34).

20

Relapse!

CLINICAL DATA—AUGUST 13, 1975: "Patient tolerated well first injection of BCG. Return in one week for second injection, plus adriamycin, Vincristine, 6MP, and prednisone."

Go, BCG! And while you're at it, rev up Kim's immunity against defeat and despair. We're counting on you. It's the seventh-inning stretch; the score is tied; you're the pinch hitter!

Dear Debbie,

Hi! How have you been? Me—so-so. Yesterday I had a blood test, spinal tap, and bone-marrow done, and am I ever so sore! And this is in between those BCG shots. I hate all that stuff with a passion!

This summer has really gone by quickly. Seems we just got out of school, and here it is fixin' to start back again.

I wish you were here, so you could give me some advice and just talk to me. It's hard to write down your feelings, on paper.

Love,
KIM

P.S. Guess what Mom and I did last week? We just packed our duds and drove to Aspen and spent a couple of days with Aunt Martha, Kathy, and Louie! It was so neat; we just stopped anywhere we wanted to along the way, picked wild flowers, went to Vail and walked around all those interesting little shops there. Had so much fun— just us girls!

(SMILE!)
KJ

September 2 FIRST DAY OF SCHOOL—ninth grade! It was only a half day, but that was plenty for me!

Came home and mom took me to the hospital for my chemotherapy. I got a feeling they don't think this BCG is doing a bit of good. I signed up for Jazz Band pianist tryouts and Poms tryouts (like cheerleaders). How's that! I don't care if that ol' BCG works or not! I'm going to beat this thing, anyway!

Kim is accelerating the ordinarily hectic pace of beginning a new school year: the extra piano practicing needed for Jazz Band auditions and accompaniment for the school choir, voice auditions for a girls' singing group, practicing the physically exhausting routines for Poms tryouts, going to Newton's after-school football games and to Arapahoes' on the weekends, running for class representative to the student council, plus the academic pressures of more difficult and demanding subjects—not to mention the weekly trips to Children's Hospital for chemotherapy and the unpredictable reactions.

September 9 Well, I made it through the first week of school, without any tremendous problems. Biology is hard.

Mom picked me up during second hour and took me to the hospital. Had blood tests, BCG, and chest X rays. Have had a nagging cough for several days.

John Beaty called tonight. He's really nice and good-looking! I'll get to see him Saturday at the Schlumberger picnic. I'm super tired tonight ZZZ!

It's only a week into September, and already my calendar of this month looks like an old doodle pad! The blocked numbers of days are barely visible through the notations of appointments and commitments to be met.

Periods of depression are the hardest to cope with. My mental energies are programmed to supporting Kim's will to live. It's an enormous juggling of my emotions. I never speak as freely as I really wish, for fear of emotional outbursts that would affect the whole family. It has happened before and is not an experience I want repeated. Even Jim and I cannot speak freely to each other anymore. His way of coping is to not confront anything, unless absolutely necessary. I respect his position only because I do not want any emotional traumas at home to jeopardize his job. So I live more and more within my own soul. It is the only place I can find the strength to survive. Solitude is my only defense. I seek it diligently and am often criticized for doing so. But the criticism doesn't even merit answering. I know its worth.

And so I create a monster, a sweeping under the rug, a delusive habit. But it is the only way I know to keep some semblance of normalcy in our lives. For emotions are like mirrors; they reflect and bounce off one another.

God, I'm no psychiatrist! Help me! What am I to say? What am I to do? It's like walking on eggshells every day, trying to keep everybody reasonably happy and productive. I need more than mere courage, God. I need perseverance and stamina. Help me not to resent, not to resist, these trying demands leukemia is imposing on my life, too. It would only increase the pain.

As days go by, the need to endure seems to increase my capacity to do so.

September 29 Guess what! I made Jazz Band! But I didn't make Poms, which is just as well. My back just killed me every time I jumped up and down. I tried, though. Anyway I get to learn how to play the electric piano for Jazz Band. The

only trouble is mom will have to take me to school at 7:00
every morning. But it will be fun. I'm working on some poster
ideas mom gave me for the Knights' Council election. Pam is
helping me, too. I hope I get it! Ate supper and worked on my
homework. I've got books running out my ears! After I finished, I popped my pills and went to bed.

Jim and I decide to have a family portrait made, outdoors, with
aspen trees in the background. An appointment is set with the
photographer for October 6.

October 6 I was late getting to school, because the bus broke
down, and they had to send another one. I made the girls'
singing group! I am really glad. We're going to make long,
checked-gingham dresses to wear. Pam was so upset today.
She found her little black kitten dead, squashed in the middle
of the street. That's so sad. I know how awful I would feel if
anything ever happened to Daisy! Got out of school at 2:00,
and the family drove to the mountains, to an aspen grove, to
have our picture taken. Mom made us get all dressed up. Jame
and I wanted to wear Levis! It was real pretty up there. I hope
it turns out nice, but we'll probably look dumb! Went to my
piano lesson after supper and played awful. This week I'm
really going to practice hard.

Kim's white blood count on October 8 is only 0.9. I begin to
see yellow, flashing lights every time I close my eyes. I am afraid
BCG is not going to be our knight in shining armor after all. The
white horse is plodding. God, I'm so afraid. I feel as if fear is the
only thing that keeps me functioning. We'll find out for sure October 16, bone-marrow day.

October 14 ELECTION DAY—I put up some more posters
early this morning. The voting was first hour. They an-
nounced who made it, over the loudspeakers, sixth hour, and

guess who did? *Me*, that's who! Those big shots can't have everything! I'm so glad I made it! The family was real proud of me. After supper I worked on homework till I couldn't stay awake anymore. I'm getting worried about my bone-marrow, Thursday.

So here we go again. October 16 finds us walking through institutional doors; down polished, tiled hallways; into steel gray elevator doors, opening in the midst of a clinical beige wall; getting out on the fifth floor; back into elevator; out on second floor; checking into the clinic; waiting for Kim's name to be called. Watching Kim walk slowly away, at the sound of her name, clutching the buckeye in her sweaty palm, I am overcome with the feeling that time is grinding slowly to a halt, as Jim and I settle into that awful, familiar, time of waiting. We can't even talk to each other. Trivia sticks in my throat. Our thoughts cautiously make their way over minefields of "what if."

At last Taru comes to the door and calls us. We get up quickly, holding our breaths. But my eyes read in her face what I refuse to hear.

The door closes behind us, in the conference room. Taru begins softly, haltingly, "I'm sorry; it's not good news. Kim has relapsed."

I don't hear any more. My Tinkertoy body is breaking apart at every joint. *Relapse*, I am paralyzed by those two syllables. The heartache is deeper this time. We know the enemy well now. We know that with each relapse, a remission becomes more difficult to obtain. The big hope, *cure*, is fading. Small, reachable hopes are our goals now.

21

Courage

October 16, 1975

Dear Debbie,

So many things have been happening since I wrote you last. Today I have to have a bone-marrow and spinal tap, so I didn't go to school. Well, mom is calling for me, and we have to be at the hospital in forty-five minutes, so I'll finish this after I get back, if I'm well enough!

Debbie, I'm so scared of these. I can remember when I was little and had to just get a shot or something, once in a while, and mom would say, "Just think, you won't have to go through this again for a whole year." And I'd always feel better, knowing that. But it's not that way at all now and never will be until I'm in heaven. It's just one continuous pain that will never leave my mind. Well, got to go.

Hi, I just got back from the hospital, and I wish I'd never gone in the first place! The results on the bone-marrow showed the leukemia has come back. Mom was teary all day, and dad kind of quiet. It makes me wonder if I know the whole story. Pam came over to cheer me up.

Love ya!

KIM

THE WEEKLY REGIMEN of L-Asparaginase begins once more. I feel as if Kim and I are in a race that everyone but the runners knows is lost. But I can't stop. And I can't let Kim stop, either. I'd rather go down biting the dust than yield to the beckoning voice of defeat!

> How do you know what is going to happen tomorrow? For the length of your lives is as uncertain as the morning fog—now you see it; soon it is gone. . . . be patient, like a farmer who waits until the autumn for his precious harvest to ripen. Yes, be patient. And take courage. . . . Job is an example of a man who continued to trust the Lord in sorrow; from his experiences we can see how the Lord's plan finally ended in good, for he is full of tenderness and mercy.
>
> James 4:14, 5:7, 8, 11

October 28—I think it is just another routine chemotherapy trip to the hospital. I should know better. Nothing in relapse is ever automatic. But I get so tired of always expecting the worst!

They have an awful time getting the needle in, even working on both arms. Each time they try, Kim screams in pain—finally, a good vein. Kim stops crying, her face so flushed and hot. She settles into a deep depression as the drug flows into her body.

Dr. Hays pushes slowly, but Kim begins to cry again. "Mother, it stings like fire going in!" Within five minutes she is violently ill. I'm struck with terror at the sight of her. Numbly I step into the hall as the emergency team rushes inside. God, I'm so scared! Jim's not here. I feel so alone and helpless.

Twenty minutes later, I catch the sounds of "crisis past" coming from Kim's room. Kim is feeling better as I reenter. Her blood pressure is still being monitored. Her face is still flushed, but she says she feels okay, as if she's floating. She starts chattering away

about nothing, then it's tears, then smiles. I know it's the Bena-
dryl.

By midafternoon we're finally able to leave. She sleeps with
her head in my lap, all the way home. Drained, absolutely
drained, both of us.

God, look in the classified section under Help Wanted. I've got
an ad: "COURAGE—to increase faith, sustain hope, face uncer-
tainties, to hang in there; reassurance of unlimited supply
needed each day. Challenging opportunity to observe certain
growth." How 'bout it, God?

> **October 28**   This day was a bummer. I got up feeling so weak
> and tired. After giving my student-council report, first hour,
> mom picked me up and we went to the hospital. After my
> blood test, I went to the clinic to get my IV medications. The
> nurse put the needle in my wrist, since my arm was so bug-
> gered up, but it leaked and got so puffed up it looked like a
> golf ball under my skin! And it hurt awfully! Then I had a bad
> reaction to the medicine, and they had to give me oxygen.
> Now I've got a huge bruise on my hand. I didn't feel good the
> rest of the day! When I got home, Pam called. Her brother
> Randy was in a car wreck and is in the hospital. I went over to
> her house, to cheer her up.

When Jim and I return from the high school's Back to School
Night for parents, Kim is watching a movie on television, based
on the life of Babe Zaharias.

"Mom, come watch this with me. She has cancer, too."

It is near the end of the movie. Kim starts crying when it is apparent that Babe Zaharias is dying. Kim buries her face in my
chest, sobbing.

"Oh, mother, I don't want that to happen to me!"

I have no words of consolation or hope, because it wasn't just a
movie. It was real. It happened. Another valiant fight against

cancer lost. It's hard for Kim not to draw comparisons. My heart is breaking again.

Everyone is asleep but Kim and me. I'm staring at the ceiling, trying to relax, trying to escape, with sleep, the throbbing ache in my heart as I listen to Kim groan. The pain in her joints is relentless, unwilling to let her rest. It is the first of many nights I am lulled into restless sleep, listening to Kim wrestle with her pain. And I can do nothing.

> Listen to my prayer, O God; don't hide yourself when I cry to you. Hear me, Lord! Listen to me! For I groan and weep beneath my burden of woe. . . . My heart is in anguish within me. Stark fear overpowers me. Trembling and horror overwhelm me. Oh, for wings like a dove, to fly away and rest! . . . I will pray morning, noon, and night, pleading aloud with God; and he will hear and answer. . . . Give your burdens to the Lord. He will carry them. . . .
>
> Psalms 55:1, 2, 4–6, 17, 22

October 31 HALLOWEEN—but this year didn't seem like Halloween at all! This was Missy's last day at school, before she moves. We gave her a party in choir, and we all started crying. Went to the football game tonight and afterwards a bunch of us went to Shakey's for pizza. Then we came back over to my house for a slumber party. Missy was sure surprised. We're eatin' popcorn and listening to records now. Probably won't get to sleep tonight!

Dawn is already pouring down the foothills, when I come downstairs to start breakfast for the girls, the next morning. I stop at the pantry door and take down the calendar, slowly turning over October's page. For the first time I don't contemplate the coming days. My fingers don't walk through the weeks, wondering what the days will bring. I smooth the page and hang the calendar back in place.

November fifth dawns crisp and clear. Soft, billowy clouds are already floating toward the mountain peaks, for a day's rest. I pick Kim up at school, at 9:15, to take her to the hospital. She comes out the side doors, all smiles. My heart skips to her joy. She had a test first period, but says it was easy. Then she just chatters away about fun things.

I haven't seen her this happy in a long time, especially en route to the hospital! Thankfulness floods my soul. She talks about how she and some friends are planning a band act for the spring talent show, wanting to play ukulele, washboard with thimble, Jew's harp, washtub bass, and so on. She's full of questions and ideas. How many times we have driven this long route together, seldom in such good spirits.

One of the two parking-metered spaces in front of the hospital is vacant. That doesn't happen very often. I take it, because we probably won't be here longer than thirty minutes. We go up to the fifth floor, and Kim gets her blood test made. Jim is waiting in the clinic, when we get back. I don't expect him, and we're very glad to see him.

"Hi, dad! Nothin' exciting going on today, but welcome to the show."

We wait for Dr. Hays in one of the small examining rooms, back in the clinic. Kim takes off her new hiking boots and puts them on the scales—three pounds. I could have sworn they weighed ten! Kim weighs herself—104 pounds.

"Boy, I don't want to get any fatter. At my age this ain't baby fat no more!"

Mary Jo and Dr. Hays come in and give Kim a brief examination, while asking her questions. Then, bombshell: They must do a bone-marrow today. Anxiety erases Kim's smiles. She begins to cry. Jim and I have to leave the room while they prepare her. We linger nervously outside the door. I want to be near Kim, yet I can't stand her cries of pain.

Suddenly Kim screams. It's not a cry of pain. It's a scream of sheer agony. Jim and I flee to the waiting room. Is there a worse sound to parents' ears than the painful, unendurable scream of their child in helpless agony?

Half an hour later we go into her room. She is sobbing. Her face is flushed and wet.

"Mom, it hurt me so badly," she whispers. "Please don't let them do it again!"

An hour later, Dr. Hays comes back. Kim is still in relapse. Mary Jo comes in to start the IV. They're going to give her L-Asparaginase and cytosine. I'm exhausted, hurting for my child so. I wish I could just lie down and turn myself off.

It's noon before we're able to leave. Jim walks us to the car. There's a parking ticket on the windshield.

Once more we're driving through downtown traffic, on our way home, Kim's head resting on the edge of my lap. Our spirits are dangerously low.

"Mom, I wonder what it would be like not to have any worries—to just be a regular kid."

> **November 11** It's still cold! Had to get up early for Jazz Band practice. School wasn't too thrilling. I feel as if I'm falling behind in all my subjects and just can't catch up. Talked to Mrs. Buckley about it. Stayed after school again for algebra, but couldn't seem to solve my problems. I'm so tired and worried. Gave Susan her piano lesson when I got home. Then we watched a TV special on the life of a boy who had leukemia. His name was Eric. He was a lot like me. And he died. I don't want to die. But, anytime, I guess I will.

It's Tuesday. Why does each day seem so precious now? I can't shake the feeling of needing to hang on to each day. My heart freezes as I walk into Kim's room to wake her for school. She looks as if she has been in a car accident. It's another nosebleed. She's had them occasionally and is worried about being embarrassed, should one occur at school. This is the worst one. Circles of dark red blood drench her pillow and sheets. She insists on going to school. She doesn't want to miss Jazz Band practice. So I stuff her coat pockets with tissues, and out she goes, trying to keep her head back. God, help my baby.

At 9:15 the school nurse calls. Kim is in the office, with a nosebleed. I am already dressed and ready to go. I call Children's and leave word that I'm bringing Kim in. God, I'm so frightened!

We have a long, close conversation all the way to Children's. Dear God, give me grace and wisdom. Help me to be calm. My heart is ripping apart, and I want to scream! Help me to concentrate on my driving. The traffic is heavy, and it's just a blur. Please keep me alert. Don't let me have a stupid wreck. Help me to be able to answer Kim's questions. Help me.

"You know we really should turn, 'Why?' around," I tell her. "Why don't we ever wonder why we've had so many years of happiness? Why don't we ever say, 'Why me, Lord, why all these years of happiness? It's such a wonderful life. Why are we never surprised at the good things that flood our lives? It's really far more remarkable that beauty should exist. That's God's original plan for his world; and suffering, pain, troubles, tragedies are all distortions of that plan, brought through man's freedom of choice. Well, anyway, it's easier to say than to accept, when one is hurting so.

"But I do know this, Kim, God loves us and is with us. We must *never* forget that."

"I know, mom."

By the time we get to the hospital, there's a pile of blood-soaked tissues on the floor of the car. Dr. Steve Dubansky meets us in the clinic. I'm so glad to see him. He has a terrific sense of humor and such rapport with the kids. Kim loves to be around him. He gets Kim into bed, takes care of the nosebleed, then calls Dr. Hays and Mary Jo.

Kim looks so pale. Mary Jo comes back with the blood count. Oh, my God: platelets—0! She doesn't have *any* platelets! WBC 0.9, hemo. 9.7, RBC 2.93. Dear God, help us. Dr. Hays calls the blood bank and tells them to send down three units of platelets. Then she calls me into a side room and asks me to sit down. I'll never forget the feel of this cold, hard, steel folding chair, because my insides feel the same way.

Taru has difficulty finding the right words. There are none. "Beth, Kim is slipping."

My face freezes in expressionless tracks. I feel like an old building being slowly and irrevocably dismantled. I cannot imagine rising again. My grief is so great.

"Kim has been talking about wanting to go to New Orleans and Houston, Beth. If you're planning such a trip, I would suggest you go as soon as possible—at least between Thanksgiving and Christmas."

Does that mean what I think it means? Oh, God. I can't hear any more. I can't cope with such thoughts. My mind flings open the cupboard of medical science, and it's bare.

22

Thou Art With Me

I FEEL I AM NOW in a constant state of prayer. Prayer is my leveler, my watermark of sanity. Bouncing back and forth from anger to submissiveness, I always know God is with me. I challenge His wisdom over and over, but I never doubt His love.

Who then can ever keep Christ's love from us? When we have trouble or calamity, when we are hunted down or destroyed, is it because he doesn't love us anymore? And if we are hungry, or penniless, or in danger, or threatened with death, has God deserted us? No, for the Scriptures tell us that for his sake we must be ready to face death at every moment of the day—we are like sheep awaiting slaughter; but despite all this, overwhelming victory is ours through Christ who loved us enough to die for us. For I am convinced that nothing can ever separate us from his love. Death can't, and life can't. The angels won't, and all the powers of hell itself cannot keep God's love away. Our fears for today, our worries about tomorrow, or where we are—high above the sky, or in the deepest ocean—nothing will ever be able to separate us from the

love of God, demonstrated by our Lord Jesus Christ when
he died for us.

Romans 8:35–39

November 21 Brrrrrrrr, the low today was one degree!
Went to school early for a ninth-grade council meeting. I got
completely exhausted today, just like yesterday. What a
bummer! Tami came over awhile tonight. Worked on my rib-
bon pillow I'm making mom for Christmas and my patchwork
quilt.

November 22 I had an awful time sleeping last night. During the night, all of a sudden, my legs had sharp aches for several minutes. Mom kept giving me Tylenol. Boy, it hurt awful
bad. Felt better this morning. Mom took me to the mall this
afternoon to get material for my next home ec. project. But I
got so tired we had to go sit down by the fountain every few
minutes.

Monday brings another snowy, cold morning. Kim is so tired,
and yet she's slowly getting ready for school. She doesn't consider staying home. Her dark eyes and wig are in stark contrast
to her pale face. She sits on the bottom stairs, leaning against the
wall, while I put on her hiking boots. My heart breaks as I watch
her go slowly down the sidewalk toward the bus stop. I go to the
kitchen window, then to the back door, to keep her in sight. She
stops and leans against our fence. God, I can't stand it any longer.
I open the back door, to call to her, but she's gone on. A chilling
breeze is blowing the swirling snow. I shut the door and collapse,
in tears. Dear God, please help my baby. She's cold and weak
and very determined to win this battle.

The phone rings as Jame comes downstairs, ready for school.
"Mrs. Jameson, this is Sheri. Kim got to my house, but she can't
walk. Please come."

Jame goes to get her. She comes in the house, crying, angry

because she's been studying for a social studies test and doesn't want to miss it. Dr. Hays suggests that I take her to school for the test, then bring her down to the hospital for transfusions. Kim agrees, but doesn't want to miss teaching her piano pupils this afternoon, either!

I wait for her in the school parking lot. Soon she comes out the cafeteria door and walks, with great effort, toward the car. I open the door for her, and her books tumble in, just ahead of her body. She looks up at me and smiles weakly.

"I made a hundred, mom! Now wasn't that worth it?"

Oh, God.

They run more tests at the hospital, and she gets typed and cross matched for the transfusions that will begin in the morning. I wonder if we will be able to make the trip to Plainview, which we are planning for Thanksgiving, only two days away. Surely, after the transfusions, Kim will feel good again.

Tuesday, November 25—It's snowing and cloudy. Kim wants to go to Jazz Band practice and take an English test before she goes to the hospital. So I take her to school at 7:30. Hold it, transfusion—got to get these important things done first!

By 10:00 we're on our way. Kim is sleeping. God, she's pale. It's going to be a long day. I packed a big Texas flag, the Neiman-Marcus Christmas catalog, and a Texas dictionary in my bag—just in case our spirits needed a break. And of course I have the buckeye.

They're waiting for us. Mary Jo saved Kim a color TV room. Here we go again. Mary Jo can't find a good vein. Over and over she tries. Kim cries out in sharp bursts of pain. God, how it tears me up to have to just stand against the wall, out of the way, and helplessly watch and listen. Her arms are so slim and white and covered with dark bruises and puncture marks. It takes nearly an hour to get a good vein and begin the transfusion process. Dr. Hays starts the L-Asparaginase first.

Suddenly Kim has a reaction to it. Her head tilts back, body jerking, guttural sounds of agony come from her half-open, blu-ish lips. As they rush oxygen to her, I flee the room. I can't stand it any longer. I call Jim. It is more than I can bear alone. God, help my baby, please.

When everything is under control, I go back to Kim's room. Oh, God, she's so still. How very pale and fragile she looks. Dark circles rim her large, dark eyes, finally at peace. Her perspiring face glistens as she whispers, with a smile, "Hi, mom."

Jim comes in. He sits beside her bed and reaches for her hand, saying very little; he just keeps stroking her fingers—those "mil-lion-dollar fingers" with the blue birthstone ring.

The packed cells and platelets arrive. It will be a long, slow process. Jim leaves to go back to the office. I walk with him to the parking lot, to get some air.

"Beth, I can't come over here again. I'm just not strong enough to take it and then go back to work. I'm sorry, I just can't. You'll have to take care of everything yourself."

So the emotional load I carry gets heavier. But I understand. I know the emotional strain, just trying to carry out normal every-day functions of running a household with the appearance of "all's well" and with a ready smile. And nothing must jeopardize his job. The small horrors of the coming days will not be shared with anyone. It is Kim and me and God.

The IVs drip in slow, steady rhythm with the big institutional clock out in the hallway, as the afternoon wears on. About three o'clock I hear Dr. Dubansky coming. Kim and I call him Bro. Steve. The lilt of his voice and laughter drifts through the halls like ringing bells.

"Kim, Bro. Steve is coming. Let's really lay Texas on him!"

A hint of excitement sparkles Kim's eyes. "Yeah, get the flag. I'll use it for a blanket."

A short time later, Bro. Steve comes in Kim's room. We're ready: The big Texas flag covers Kim and the bed; she's reading the Texas dictionary; I have my feet propped up, reading the

Neiman-Marcus Christmas catalog! Bursts of laughter break out, simultaneously. Kim asks him to read the Texas dictionary to us, in his New Jersey accent. The heavy atmosphere of this room suddenly changes, as the hilarity draws others. God, thank You for laughter. Thank You for a sense of humor. Thank You for this moment that lifts our spirits so. Thank You.

It is six o'clock before the IVs are finished and we can go home. Even with the gloomy prognosis, I feel that Kim will begin to get better now. Always, before, transfusions have given her new life. We decide to go ahead with our plans for a Texas Thanksgiving.

Wednesday, November 26—Kim is playing "The Entertainer" on the piano, while I load the car. Although I do not know it, it is to be the last time I will hear her play. She will not come home again. By midmorning, Kim and I and Daisy are ready to leave for Plainview. The sun is shining, but the streets and highways are icy. I'm apprehensive about driving the more than five hundred miles that stretch ahead of us, but our relatives are expecting us and planning a big reunion. Kim is so looking forward to the trip, that I know we must go. And we need the good times that a family reunion always brings. Jim and Jame will follow us, after Jim gets home from work this evening.

Thanksgiving Day, Plainview, Texas—Jim and Jame arrived safely about three-thirty in the morning. Kim has not slept well and is restless this morning.

"Mom, I'm so tired. And I don't feel good. When am I going to feel better? Wasn't I supposed to feel better after the transfusions?"

Icy apprehension begins to grip me. Yes, she should be feeling good by now, having had three units of platelets, two of packed red cells, and L-Asparaginase. I don't understand. The pain in her joints is increasing. She's even having difficulty walking. She dresses slowly, then rests on the divan.

"Maybe you just need some good ol' turkey and dressing, with all the trimmin's," I tell her.

But after eating very little, Kim goes into a back bedroom and lies down. When I check her, she is running a fever. That awful hollow feeling of fear sweeps over me as Jim and I excuse ourselves and put in a call to Dr. Hays. Taru tells us to keep giving her Tylenol and, if the fever doesn't go down in a few hours, call her back. God, Kim feels awful. I hurt, too. I think I know more than my mind is accepting.

I'm having a hard time being thankful to You, God. How can I be happy and thankful for all Your blessings, for all the good things of life we're supposed to be recalling today, when I am so saddened? I don't feel thankful at all, God. I really feel angry. Why does Kim have to suffer so?

By evening Kim's fever is down, so I decide not to call Taru back. Maybe by morning she will be better. I climb into bed with Kim; we both drift off into a restless sleep, but not for long. In the silence of the night, I'm alert to Kim's voice.

"Mom, I hurt all over. There's no place I can move that I don't have awful pain."

I reach over to hold her, pat her forehead—anything.

"Don't, mom, don't touch me. Every place on my body just hurts too much for you to even touch me."

"Kim, baby—"

I'm paralyzed with fear as she continues in a soft, trembling voice, "Mom, I want to tell you something, and I don't want you to feel bad or anything. But I want God to take me on to heaven. I just can't stand this pain any longer. I've just been lying here thinkin', and that's what I've decided. No one can feel this bad and be the least bit well. I believe I'm on the homestretch to heaven. Let's pray, Mom. I love you."

The pain is so great that she slips in and out of consciousness, uttering indescribable sounds of agony. Her lips are blue, her eyes rolling to the back of her head—telling the intensity of her pain, as no words can.

Dear God, please don't let her die—not now, not here! I am frantic to get back to Denver. It is our last, desperate hope.

With more codeine, she gradually eases; and Jim begins calling airlines, for a flight to Denver. Then we start packing. Jim and Jame leave in the car, with Daisy, by 3:30 A.M. I will take a flight, with Kim, out of Lubbock, at 8:45 A.M. We should arrive in Den- · ver about the same time.

Getting Kim's Levis on and raising her arms to put her shirt on is an agonizing accomplishment.

Thank goodness the plane is on time. She's gritting her teeth and trembling all over as the flight attendants carry her on board. They put us in first class, so Kim will be more comfortable. I'm so grateful. Come on, flight 253, get us to Denver quickly and safely. You're a part of our miracle now. We need you! Fear sweeps over my dry, parched soul like a prairie fire on a windy day, devouring every seedling of hope that struggled to survive.

We'll be in Denver soon.

As we approach, the plane suddenly breaks through the clouds, revealing a breathtaking view of the Rocky Mountain Range, glistening in the sunshine of a brand-new day. My God, the earth is riddled with Your divinity. How can it be overlooked so much! Even in my grief, I can see Your majestic powers at · work. Lord, I release my child to You. Help me to accept what lies ahead. Help Jame and Jim as they are driving. They haven't had any sleep. Oh, God, help us through this day! We're Yours. The Lord is my Shepherd. . . . Yea, though I walk through the valley of the shadow of death, I will fear no evil: for thou art with me. . . . Thou art with me. . . . *Thou art with me*. . . .

23

Angel Unaware

CHILDREN'S HOSPITAL, DENVER.

November 30   Today I've had news I had been dreading. They only have maybe two drugs left that can possibly help me. If not, I'm just going over this headboard to head out for heaven. I really thought I'd beat this thing. I've tried so very hard! But I must have done something wrong—I don't know what. From my window, I can see into the windows of the newborn center, in the next wing. I think about what they're doin' over there, and all those brand-new babies just startin' to live. I sure do pray that they will be healthy and strong. I hope none of them will ever have anything as bad as leukemia. This writing is awful, because I'm so tired. I can't write so well anymore.

By late afternoon, Kim's school friends begin streaming in. She wants the door shut, so she'll be sure to have her wig on when someone comes—and lipstick, too! Leukemia is an endless invasion of dignity. She wages a battle of self-worth, because of it. And looking her best is part of winning.

Flowers, plants, cards, posters begin filling the room—symbols of love, friendship, and prayers from her many friends. God, her life has touched so many, in so little time!

Her homemaking teacher brings letters from her classmates, expressing such thoughts as: "Your sweet spirit has made a lasting impression on my life." "You're really a good friend, Kim. Everyone misses you and is praying for you." "Kim, I never thought about death, before, until you got sick. I've always thought it just happened to old people and people you didn't know. I think about it now. And I'm changing my ways about a lot of things that are wrong with my life. I hope I can be more like you. God bless you."

A bed is brought in, so I can stay with Kim at night. Jim stays until we're both ready for sleep. He tucks the sheet around Kim's shoulder and places L'il Darlin'—the teddy bear Pam brought Kim Sunday night—against the bed rail. Jim kisses her goodnight.

"I'll see you in the morning, babe."

As I read his grieving eyes, I know we are both thinking the same thing. Each time we say good-night, is it for the last time? Each day, we are all living a little and dying a little.

I cling to the moments alone in the dark with Kim, after her father and brother leave for the night. It's a time of sharing our thoughts and observations on what is happening. At the same time, I fear them for statements she makes that tear my heart to shreds. And I need to react calmly to anything she says. She is becoming so sensitive to my feelings. It is hardly the same mother-daughter special sharing times we spent in her canopy bed. There is no trivia in these conversations. It is conversation between mother and dying daughter. The fact that she is so aware makes these times even more painful.

"How much time do I have, mom? What's the most? What did Dr. Hays say was the least? Did Mrs. Randal really say I was a good Christian influence at school?"

Tears stream softly down my face and I fight to keep my voice steady. Staring at the ceiling, I embroider memories around each word Kim speaks.

"Mom, it's occurred to me that I might not get well at all—
ever. Any time I was sick before, I was always thinking, 'Now
when I get well, I'm going to do this and that . . . ,' and how I was
going to catch up on all the stuff I missed, being sick. Getting
well always followed getting sick. But that's not true, is it? Sometimes dying follows being sick. You know, I think that's what's
happening to me, mom. I think I'm dying, and I'm scared. I know
I'll be in heaven, but I'm scared of getting there. And I'm confused, because I'm just a kid. . . . I'm not ready yet. There's so
much livin' left to do, mom."

Oh, God, what can I say? The agonizing pain of my aching
heart is overwhelming. Give me control and wisdom to help my
child. Sleep is merciful, but does not come easily. I lie in the dark
a long time, suffering silently, listening to the sounds of Kim's
painful, restless sleep.

It's late, and I'm standing beside Kim's bed as she restlessly
sleeps. The street light casts its reflections over Kim's bed, in the
darkness. She mumbles and talks occasionally of remote subjects. I'm dying piecemeal. This child is so much a part of my existence. My body is raked raw with unimagined heartbreak, as I
search her flawless face, glistening in the dark. Dear God, is she
an angel unaware?

"Mom, where are you and dad going to have my funeral?"

My heart stops, as I rigidly turn around to face her.

"I was just thinkin' about my funeral. Oh, I don't know. I don't
really want to think about it yet. Read me the Twenty-third
Psalm again. . . ." She drifts off.

God, oh, my God, help me to be brave. I sit beside her and
read the Psalm. It's her favorite, and she seems to derive great
comfort from hearing it each time.

"Mom, you know I don't think I have been a very good witness for Christ. I don't think my Christianity has been very ef-
fective." She smiles at my reassurance and closes her eyes again,

tears tracking her feverish cheeks.

Oh, God, are You *sure* You need her more than I do?

"Mom, I've been thinking about all the letters and what my friends are thinking about their relationships to God. And, well, if my dying helps them to know what it means to be Christians, then it's okay; I'll do it."

"Will I get to see PauPau [Kim's grandfather]? Is Grannie Ruth coming soon? Give my special things to Pam and Debbie. Be sure to give Pam my Bible. I want Jame to have my savings account, to help him at college next year. I still don't understand it, mom: Why Christians have to suffer and die. Looks to me like the Lord could use more of us here on earth! Well, I knew it was going to happen. That night in Plainview, God told me. He told me I was on the homestretch to heaven. I'm going to try to go to sleep, but it sure is hard, when I'm hurting so badly. I'm ready to say my prayers."

Twenty-eight months of fighting you, leukemia, has not left us as unprepared for this final skirmish as you may think. Spiritual roots have grown deep, adapting to nature's demands for survival, ready to give sustenance as all other sources of help begin to fail. Those roots allow the growth of new shoots of courage, when others break off from the weight of anguish and grief.

> . . . When the great oak is straining in the wind,
> The boughs drink in new beauty, and the trunk
> Sends down a deeper root on the windward side.
> Only the soul that knows the mighty grief
> Can know the mighty rapture. Sorrows come
> To stretch out spaces in the heart for joy.
>   EDWIN MARKHAM

So you see, you still won't be victorious, even though you unleash death—your final blow—because the Resurrection of Jesus Christ stands as the vindication of God's intent to destroy death once and for all. Even though we are stunned with sorrow, we are united with God, and life is a continuation. It is not—as you would like us to believe, in your evil guise of leukemia—*the end!*

Oh, my God, how dark is this hospital room! Are You *ever* coming back with the light of understanding, or must we continue to trust in the dim light of acceptance? Though my soul is in anguish, use this time of darkness to strengthen my faith. Teach me the meaning of blind trust. Achieve life's purpose, for Your eye is on the whole of this conflict. As the weaver on life's loom, You are working from above and can see it all. You know what the finished product will be. But I am on the bottom, looking up. Nothing looks right. It's tangled threads, mismatched patterns, colors going berserk in all pointless directions on the shuttle of time. It will only be when the weaving stops and the tapestry of my life is turned that I will see the real worth and purpose of it all. I'm below "see level," God. Lead me through this dense thicket of questioning, for I'm blinded with grief. But I know—*I know*—You are on the other side!

> This body is my house—it is not I;
> Herein I sojourn till, in some far sky,
> I lease a fairer dwelling, built to last
> Till all the carpentry of time is past . . .
> This body is my house—it is not I.
> Triumphant in this faith I live . . . and die.
> "The Tenant"
> FREDERICK L. KNOWLES

Dawn breaks abruptly through the darkness, wrapping up my world, again taking up preparations to give a glorious present back to God.

Wednesday, December 3—another day, another precious day of twenty-four clinging, clutching hours. How many have I let pass so frivolously? How passively they slip away when one is living.

How alarming is the speed when one is dying.

It's 7:00, and the morning sun is beginning to fill the room. I quietly close the blinds, for Kim is finally resting well.

The sound of her soft voice startles me, "Mom, my toes are the only things that don't hurt. I'm trying hard to just think of my toes. Mama, oh, mama, I hurt so much that I just want to go on to heaven. Is that wrong? I wish I could go without pain, but I guess it's not going to be that way. I've just had too much of it."

The day passes haltingly, as more flowers and mail arrive, more gifts and friends doing their best to cheer and encourage. But it's a day of erratic emotions. For, as soon as the door closes and we're alone, Kim sobs with the torture of her pain, unable to control, behind a smile, its intensive raging throughout her body.

I take off her wig and wipe her perspiring face and head with a cool, damp towel. She drifts off into an exhausted state of rest. I pull up a chair beside her bed and rest my head against the coolness of her slim fingers. My soul is already flooding with an intolerable sense of loss.

"Mom, have you and dad decided where to have my funeral?"

Grief-laden shoulders raise my sorrow-lined face to meet the gaze of my almost-fifteen-year-old daughter. The shock of her question engulfs me once more.

"It's okay, mom. I don't want to talk about it, either—another time . . . maybe. . . ."

My heart stops as I continue to listen.

"Do you know what's going on, mom? Do you know why I'm suffering so much? I just want to be a teenager. Is that too much? Oh, I hurt so badly! I hurt all over! I'm so tired—so tired. I want to go to heaven now, mom."

"Kim. *Kim!*"

I run to the nurse's station to call Dr. Hays. "Talk to her, Taru. She wants to die!"

Hope, however modest, had always been our primary weapon. It was a way of dividing Kim's illness into manageable portions.

Hope fortified confrontations with the harshness of realities. It was the first to arrive at the scene of battle. I embraced its coming. Now I lament its passing.

Taru finally comes out of Kim's room. "Beth, she's just given up. She knows everything medically possible has been done. I've seen it happen to teenagers over and over, when they know their disease is out of control and death is imminent. They know they are going to die, and they get tired of the struggle."

I shut the door behind her and walk stoically to Kim's bed, praying for courage and divine wisdom to heal my child's dying spirit. As I reach for Kim's hand, the assurance of God's reality is stronger than ever. My beautiful, courageous daughter has been a warrior too long. I cannot watch her leave the scene of battle a beggar. She must remain a warrior.

And thus begins a prayerful and professional "offering up" of suffering for God to use.

> Dark and repulsive though it is, suffering has been revealed to us as a supremely active principle for the humanization and divinization of the universe. Here is the ultimate meaning of the prodigious spiritual energy born on the cross ... a possible Christification of suffering. That is the miracle which has been renewed for 2000 years. The world is an immense groping, an immense search. It can only progress at the cost of many failures and much pain. The sufferers, whatever the reason for their suffering, are the reflection of this austere yet noble condition. They are not useless. They are soldiers who have fallen on the field of honor.
>
> TEILHARD DE CHARDIN

The conversation that follows between mother and daughter tears at the roots of my existence, as together we explore the inexorable path. Together we wrestle with the awesome fears of existence and nonexistence. Together we explore our little broken-toy happinesses in the light of Christ's treasure of everlasting life. And together, through instinctive petitions of prayer, we gain a measure of peace—assurance that, with Christ, even the great enigma of death can be faced victoriously.

"What is death?" Kino asked.

"Death is the great gateway," Kino's father said. His face was not at all sad. Instead it was quiet and happy.

"The gateway—where?" Kino asked again.

Kino's father smiled. "Can you remember when you were born?"

Kino shook his head. "I was too small."

Kino's father laughed. "I remember it very well. Oh, how hard you thought it was to be born! You cried and you screamed."

"Didn't I want to be born?" Kino asked. This was very interesting to him.

"You did not," his father told him, smiling. "You wanted to stay just where you were in the warm, dark house of the unborn. But the time came to be born, and the gate of life opened."

"Did I know it was the gate of life?" Kino asked.

"You did not know anything about it and so you were afraid of it," his father replied. "But see how foolish you were! Here we were waiting for you, your parents, already loving you and eager to welcome you. And you have been very happy, haven't you?"

"Until the big wave came," Kino replied. "Now I am afraid again because of the death that the big wave brought."

"You are only afraid because you don't know anything

about death," his father replied. "But someday you will wonder why you were afraid, even as today you wonder why you feared to be born."

from *The Big Wave*
Pearl S. Buck

Smiling, Kim reaches out for me with faltering arms, pressing my face gently to hers.

"Mom, when God is ready for me, I'm goin'. Okay?"

My mind zigzags through the minefield of hours that remains of this day. It is a race to reach tomorrow without my heart being blown to bits.

December 4—the worst night yet is finally over, and my child is still alive. I gaze at Kim's quiet, sallow face, glistening with perspiration from efforts to deal with her pain. Exhaustion creeps into every distant part of my body as I watch her erratic breathing. For a moment I withdraw into a comforting place of cramped nonexistence behind my opened eyes, as if to insulate myself from the predictable unfolding of events. It is a quiet moment of being fixed in a faded sepia photograph, before being interrupted by those who will make our tragedy supportable.

It is a day that marks the beginning of good-byes: good-bye to Kim's spirit of adventure, good-bye to her indomitable courage, good-bye to her inexhaustible love of life.

December 4 Well, I'm still here in the hospital. I've got a pretty nice room though, with two big windows.

It snowed when I first came here, but it's all disappeared now. It takes someone mighty, like God, to create such beautiful objects.

" 'Fight, Warriors, fight . . . ,' I never can remember all the words to Arapahoe's fight song. Mama, what did Dr. Hays say this morning? I'm not in very good shape, right? You know what, mama? I think I'm dying. That's what I think. And you know something else? It's okay. I want to talk to you; don't let me forget what I want to say. I can't remember things so well anymore. Oh, mama, I love you."

Jim comes as the breakfast tray is brought in. Jame comes as soon as his morning classes are over. Throughout the day, we all notice a definite change in Kim's spirit and attitude. The whys and flashes of anger are being replaced by the purest expressions of love and acceptance I have ever witnessed. Her heart seems bursting with gratitude at every manifestation of the thoughtfulness that literally pours into her room all day. The tapping on her door is constant, keeping her busy giving out her love to the many friends who keep coming to spend a few minutes with her. Smiles fill the room as teenage humor and news of school activities dominate the conversations. But as good-byes are said and the door is quietly closed, those smiles dissolve into heartbreaking sobs in the hall.

Kim's demonstrative outpouring of love toward everyone she comes in contact with makes me feel that this angel unaware of ours is in the process of being fitted with a new set of wings.

This evening Kim has some private good-byes to say to Pam and to Jame. They are sacred moments, not meant to be shared.

As Jame comes out in the hall, sobbing uncontrollably, Kim calls after him, "Jame, I love you, I love you Jame. Jame? I love you."

"Why her, mom? Why not me? Kim has always been the good one—so sweet, so thoughtful, and so faithful to the church, so anxious to always do what's right. She's been such a witness, especially to me. God, take me instead, please!" There is no comforting my son.

How easy it is to tell someone to "have courage, keep your faith, don't despair, time heals," when we have nothing at stake. The point of our belief comes when we have lost the battle.

While we are being pulled through the quicksand of grief and separation, death's diminishing is simultaneously firmly welding our family's connection with God. The comfort of continuation is already at work, searching for the fragments of our spirits.

Friends and relatives begin leaving, as Kim's exhaustion becomes apparent. Jim and Jame reluctantly say good-night, and Kim and I prepare for another long, restless night. Grief and logic, despair and reality are locked in fierce combat in my mind, as the inevitability of Kim's oncoming death consumes my physical and emotional energies. I kiss my child good-night, and pray that it isn't good-bye.

24

Returning to Perfection

"MOM, HOW MUCH LONGER UNTIL MORNING?"

A crack in the bathroom door releases a wedge of light across Kim's bed. Her forehead glistens with perspiration. My child, my baby, no longer has that little-girl look. Pain has matured her face. The vitality of youth is gone.

The palms of my hands receive my bowed head once more. My God, You said not one sparrow would fall to the ground without Your noticing. Are You noticing? Something beautiful, of far more value than a sparrow, is falling. Over here, God!

Blunt and childish though my continuous prayers be, they make it possible for me to accept the unacceptable. I am learning a lesson about faith, that it offers us no protection against anxiety and sorrow. But faith does offer security *in* anxiety and sorrow.

Kim wakens. "Mom, when I doze off, I dream the weirdest things. And I start wondering why all over again."

Only in the throes of pain that sweep Kim in and out of consciousness do the fragmented questions arise. "Mom, do you think I can make it to Christmas? It's only about two weeks, isn't it? That's not very far away, is it? Aren't we already in December? I just want to be at home with the family again. Maybe I'll make it, but I don't know how much more of this pain I can stand. And if I don't make it, next Christmas and all the other Christmases would remind you of what happened *this* Christmas. Oh, mom—"

Kim seems to be suspended in a body ready to die, but unwilling to die. Yesterday she couldn't wait for life. And now life can't wait for her. What a difference a day makes. . . . My world crackles with grief as it shrivels up and freezes around me.

Death, don't you have a shred of dignity? Life has rules, why don't *you*? It's just not natural for my child to suffer such a slow, agonizing, painful, irreversible illness and to die! You're supposed to wait until life has accomplished its contributing years, slowly preparing one for your coming—a climax to a task well done. You're supposed to give patience and acceptance time to grow. And, besides, children are not supposed to die before their parents do! This sudden indiscriminate snatching is deplorable! Why can't you go by the rules? Why can't you just go away until deteriorating old age welcomes your presence?

Learning how to lose a gift of love is a great challenge indeed.

At last sunlight begins to fill Kim's room. Thank You, God! How precious the hours are! Jim opens the door. My sister Martha is with him. Kim's face lights up. She's so happy to see them both, and especially their bag of doughnuts. We proceed to have a doughnut-breakfast picnic on Kim's bed! Laughter is heard once more.

The steady stream of visitors and phone calls begins early. Kim meets them all with cheerfulness and outward optimism. As the day passes, she shares her precious gift of time willingly and at great cost. It seems terribly important to her that she not miss a single opportunity to tell everyone who comes how much she loves them and how much God is loving and caring for her in this experience of suffering. In this unique way she has the grace to deal with her ceaseless pain, hour by hour. The glory of God is brilliant as she witnesses to us all. God's grace is sufficient to meet my child's needs. It is a gift beyond courage.

In a rare, quiet moment that afternoon, with only Jim and me in the room, Kim begins to move her head from side to side on her pillow, and tears stream down her face.

"Oh, mama, I'm so happy. You know Debbie, that pretty nurse? I witnessed to her. I asked her if she was a Christian and if she believed in God. Then I asked her if she believed that Jesus was God's Son and died on the cross for you and me. And she said yes! Then we prayed for each other. Debbie had to go home; she was through working. But I know I'll see her again in heaven. I'm going to share this with Pam, too. Oh, mom, dad, my prayers are answered, and I'm so happy. All these people who are coming to see us and calling—people are just so nice. I just don't deserve it!"

Jim puts his arms around us as I press my face against her flushed cheeks. It is a peaceful moment of balanced emotions that recommits our trust to the wisdom of God.

The facts of her life are closing down as Kim struggles against the process of separating herself from the body that has so impeded her. She struggles because she is not through loving and saying good-bye to those who keep coming. Jim, Jame, and I stand by as Kim's strength wanes with the hours.

The girl who first pulled off Kim's wig at school comes. She brings Kim a gold music box. Gently they embrace. It is a touching moment of love and forgiveness.

By evening, Kim is exhausted and drifts in and out of consciousness.

"My back, oh, my back. Mom please rub my back. No, don't help me. I've got to reach that railing myself. Can't 'never could' do anything!"

With intense effort, she struggles to turn on her side. Her gaunt, bruised arms reach for the metal bed railing.

"There! Thank you for that extremely well-done back rub! Hi, Jame. Jame, I love you. Pam? Are you still here? I love you, Pam. I want you to have my Bible. Now you take it and read that thing, you hear? 'Cause it's the truth.''

Jim and I sit, transfixed, on the edge of that rollaway bed, watching our child say good-bye on her own terms, to those who have enriched her life. The impending death of one's child makes a mother more aware of life than the moment of that child's birth. I was thinking about life in terms I'd never seriously considered before: its meaning; its brevity; the perspective of "things"; emphasis on today, instead of the taken-for-granted tomorrows. An impossibility had become a reality. Life and death are woven in very close patterns. I nervously pull a hang-nail too far into my cuticle. My finger throbs with pain. I am glad. Numb with grief, it is the only sensation my body can feel.

It is getting late now, but the family is hesitant to leave. I stand at the window, staring across at the newborn center, remembering what Kim had said when we first arrived at the hospital. Oh, my God, the pain my child brought me as she came into this world was great. But nothing can be compared to the pain I feel at watching her go! Surely winter has never stood so still.

A gentle tapping, and the door opens once more. It is Art Gore. I can't believe it. Once more this gentle man comes into our lives. Kim is elated as she suddenly recognizes him. He walks directly to her bed.

"Mr. Gore, is it really you? Oh, thank you for coming!"

He sits at the foot of her bed as he unwraps a package. "I brought you something, Kim. See this book? *Images of Yesterday,''* he reads. "Now let me show you the inside-cover page. There's a gold seal that says 'first edition,' and above that I've written, 'To my beautiful friend, Kim—number one of seventy-five hundred copies—December fifth, nineteen hundred seventy-five—Children's Hospital.' It's my first book. The copies just arrived from the publisher. I wanted you to have the first one.''

Kim begins to cry. "Thank you, oh, thank you so much. I never forgot the time you showed us around your studio! I love you, I love you so much, Mr. Gore. Thank you."

His voice breaks as he says good-bye. "Be back tomorrow night, Kim. I promise you that."

She can no longer suppress her suffering, as the pressure within the bone marrow screams into the megaphone of pain. Jim decides to stay with me this night. I need him. I am afraid. We push the rollaway alongside Kim's bed. In the darkness we sit, praying, crying, and watching Kim, in a restless state of sleep, slowly begin the process of disentangling herself from this life. Her image in the dimness of a night-light is being branded into my memory. Eyes closed, her head nestles comfortably in the folds of the Raggedy Ann and Andy pillowcase from her bed at home. Her face is a white shade of pale. On the table rests the buckeye. My eyes do not dwell on the massive bruises on Kim's arms, due to platelet failure. I see only my child in the process of returning to perfection.

"Mom?" Kim's soft voice penetrates the silence. Our eyes meet in a loving gaze. She smiles. "Mom, good ol' mom. Next to God, you're number one."

25

The Valley of the
Shadow of Death

DECEMBER 6—the hours of the night dwindle into dawn. It is another quiet, suspended period of time. Suddenly I awaken from watchful sleep. My eyes bolt toward Kim. She is still breathing. I hear a slight moaning. I gaze intently at my child and softly quote the Twenty-third Psalm.

"Thanks, mom," Kim whispers, her eyes still closed. Dr. Hays comes in shortly after seven-thirty, but Kim talks very little. Her voice is considerably weakened. Taru does not have to tell us that Kim is loosening her moorings to this life.

In quiet resignation, I join Kim in the direction of acceptance, though not as willingly as she. And in so doing, I feel as if I have been allowed on the inside, to wait with her in this timeless void between life and death. It is as if we are together again in a waiting room. Her name will soon be called. She will go. I will stay behind. In going, Kim's spirit will finally emerge, free and unencumbered. And those of us left behind will be unbelievably rich.

Dying, like birth, is terribly hard.

Kim, sometimes, in watching you go—however great the struggle—I think of you as being more alive now than before you had leukemia. Because, having faced death, you know what it

really means to be alive. For so many people, that interim between life and death remains insignificant. It took you only
slightly less than fifteen years to discover its worth and realize
that its true value is in giving it away.

Suddenly Kim begins coughing with deep, guttural sounds, as
if she had a bad chest cold. Her body heaves, trying to spit it out.
I reach for a towel and hold it under her lips. It isn't sputum. It is
blood.

"It's okay, honey, go ahead and get it out," I say calmly. I am
glad her eyes are closed. What the towel didn't absorb, flowed
between my fingers. God, that's my child's *life* spilling through
my fingers, like sifting sand! And I'm powerless to stop it.

"That makes me so mad," Kim says disgustedly, choking on
each word.

Thankfully, the hemorrhaging stops. I wash her face and teeth,
and she begins to relax a little.

Opening her dark, receding eyes, Kim smiles. "Mom, I'm
going to go see Paupau, and he and I are going to have a real
good time."

And then she retreats to her waiting room, imprisoned in a reality where life and death are meshed together.

Then Almitra spoke, saying, We would ask now of Death.
And he said:
You would know the secret of death.
But how shall you find it unless you seek it in the heart of life?
The owl whose night-bound eyes are blind unto the day cannot unveil
    the mystery of light.
If you would indeed behold the spirit of death, open your heart wide
    unto the body of life.
For life and death are one, even as the river and the sea are one.
                                                        KAHLIL GIBRAN

All of us in this room are witnesses to the culmination of perfection. Life and death are in complete harmony. The family cir-

cle grows closer. Taru, Mary Jo, clinic nurses who had fought the battle so valiantly with us, are coming now, to give their support as friends. Once inside our room, they step out of their professional roles to complete the circle of love surrounding Kim's bed. In a sense, their tears are more anguished than ours. For with theirs are mingled dashed hopes and bitter frustrations. Brilliantly they directed the battle plan, but now the supply of weapons is exhausted. Knowledge without tools is useless.

Doris Lund, the author of *Eric*, the story of her son's fight with leukemia, was right. A hospital is both a heaven and a hell. The hell is obvious. The heaven is created by the people who work there.

Darkness falls softly past our windows, like crumpled velvet, snuffing out the light of Kim's last day on earth. The flickering lights of the city multiply, turning on in sequence, as if one long string of Christmas lights. The whole world outside this window seems alive, but me. The atmosphere of this room reeks of an abandoned carnival, as silence and muffled cries replace joy and laughter. Life is replacement. Death is abandonment.

I glance up as the door opens once more. My mind is hazy and irritated at being talked into taking a tranquilizer.

I suddenly recognize who it is working his way to Kim's bed. It is Art Gore, keeping his promise of the night before.

"Kim, *Kim.* Please come back. Look, it's Art Gore. He came to see you again, just as he promised. And he brought you something. Open your eyes—look, baby."

The luminous pallor of Kim's face matches the coolness of her skin as I press my hands to her cheeks. She flashes intermittent smiles as I talk, as if trying to decide whether to come back, or to continue her journey. Gently I raise her eyelids with my thumbs. I am momentarily stunned by the gaze that meets mine. Her eyes are deep, dark pools of remoteness.

"Kim, look, baby, it's an old Raggedy Ann doll—the one in Mr. Gore's picture. He wants you to have the doll. Kim?"

Her eyes gradually focus as she makes a faltering attempt to hold the doll. I tuck it into the bend of her arm. Her chin rests peacefully on the doll's faded yarn hair.

"Thank you," Kim whispers with a flickering smile. She closes her eyes once more and continues her journey.

Art Gore gently holds her hand as he talks to her. But his voice breaks as he realizes Kim is not responding. Her imprisoned spirit is ready to be freed.

Coma, death's sleeping twin, is leading my child from life into death. She doesn't answer. She is too busy dying.

I study Kim's face—the remote translucence, the spiritual radiance—and it gradually dawns on me that the love for her Saviour and her quest for heaven far surpass the love for her family and friends. The hopes and dreams and plans she held so dear are fast fading in importance.

Oh, Kim, my child, as my eyes and fingertips search your face in death, was it only fourteen years and nine months ago that I examined your face just as I'm doing now? Then I searched each tiny feature of your pink newly born face with sensitive eyes and fingers, and my heart overflowed with awe at the beautiful baby in my arms—this God-given gift, so fresh from heaven's home. And though my heart is now full of unspeakable sadness, as I trace your features once more, I am still in awe at being blessed with your presence in my life for as long as fourteen years and nine months. Your chilled face has turned from pink to gray, but there is a beautiful radiance as you "let go and let God have his wonderful way." I know it's time for me to let go also, but my grief at watching you leave is so intense!

Kim, I am haunted by the many ways I failed you. Perhaps I tried too hard to be a good mother. You were so much like me. So many times I was harsh and impatient with you over trivial matters. Remember when you ruined my last good pair of panty hose by wearing them to school, and I didn't know it until it was time to get ready to go to church? And when you left my new eye shadow open on the windowsill in the bathroom, and the sun melted it? When you wore my new green shoes that just matched a top you had made; and, when you came home, the heels were all scuffed? Remember when you'd be in a hurry to go somewhere and leave handfuls of your beautiful, long, brown hair, which was falling out, in the bathroom sink and loose strands all over the floor? Losing your glasses at school? Remember when you forgot a book you needed for a class report and called me from school to ask me to bring it to you, and I was already late for a dental appointment? When you got involved with what I considered too many extracurricular activities at school, which drained your physical strength? Just irritations over trivia! Forgive me, Kim. You were only anxious to get on with living.

Remember the pact we made at the very beginning? In your room, piled with boxes and the disorganization that comes from just moving in, we hugged each other and, with tears streaming down our faces, vowed we would never give in or give up? Oh, there were many times when each of us could not live up to this: times when you were so ill; when you were out of remission; when you were not responding properly to the drugs; when you were getting behind in your schoolwork, pushing yourself even to go to school at all. Yes, alone we let down at times, but together we remained strong. Forgive me for having loved you too much and forgetting that you and Jame are merely on loan to your daddy and me.

Oh, my God, hang on to me, for my spirit wants to let go too. I don't have the desire or right to live beyond the years of my child. How can this be? Surely it is the most unnatural of all disasters!

Kim is no longer struggling to survive. Her body is abdicating peacefully. Dying was agony. Death is gentle.

Her clasp on the Raggedy Ann doll relaxes. She slips from my arms, passing by the sting of death as one unnoticed, seeing only the face of the One who is the Resurrection and the Life.

Epilog

Dear Mr. and Mrs. Jameson,

How can I express how I feel? Kim meant so much to me. It is so hard to lose a beautiful person like Kim; but when God gave her to us, He never promised that she'd be with us forever. It's hard to accept; but through prayer, I have found help. I am so happy that Kim led me to Christ. Life means so much more now. It's wonderful that she did that for me. Kim and I shared so many beautiful moments together, and I'm so thankful I had the opportunity to know her and love her.

The first time Kim ever talked to me about God was soon after we had become friends. We were up at Woolco, looking at the jewelry. Out of nowhere Kim asked me if I believed in God. I said, no, because there were so many scientific facts that disproved the Bible. Religion was just something people turned to for reassurance and comfort. Who had ever seen or talked to God? Because God wasn't there for me to see, I didn't believe. Looking at the watches, she began to explain her belief to me. Just because I didn't understand how the watch worked or know who had made it, that didn't mean I didn't or couldn't believe the watch worked. I'm not quite sure how she put it, and there was more, but from that time on I began to look differently at religion. It has changed my life. I love you.

PAM

Dear Jameson Family,

We wanted you to know what an inspiration your daughter has been to every member of our family. We came to love Kim through church. She helped develop in Maureen and the other children a real sensitivity toward everything around her. She was so aware of other people and their feelings, of nature, flowers, and so on. Kim was full of life, even when she was so ill. She talked, laughed, and teased you, to cheer you up, when you were feeling down, and yet, inside, she knew her body was dying, inch by inch, of cancer.

We shall always be thankful for the weekend Kim spent with our family, in the mountains, last November. I could hardly believe the maturity Kim displayed for her age. At one point the kids were all hiking, and Kim needed to rest, so she and Scott sat on a fallen log, and she asked Scott if he had ever heard that every snowflake was different. He had, but never thought about it. "Well," she said, "it's very important. First, because we are like snow-flakes, we are each one different. Some snowflakes are beautiful, and some of us are beautiful. Some are perfect, and some of us are perfect; some are not perfect, and some of us are not perfect. But God decides who will be beautiful and who will be ordinary. He decides who will be perfect and who will not be perfect. God loves each one of us, and He makes us to be the way He wants us. That is why I like the snow so much, because it reminds me that we are all different—no two alike—we are exactly the way God wants us. Even if our bodies are not perfect, He loves us." Later I noticed Kim staring out the front window, with tears much larger than any snowflake, and she turned to me and said, "Mrs. Mellecker, you don't know just how beautiful that really is." I realized Kim was looking through the eyes of limited time and all I could do was cry with her and love her.

Kim glowed with the Spirit of God, for all to see, and I'm sure the six of us aren't the only ones who have changed lives because of having known Kim. She knew Him in a way that I saw and wanted also. Kim was no ordinary child, but a chosen child of God. Through her suffering, many people have come to know Christ. She truly fought the good fight.

The night our family visited her in the hospital was a night we'll never forget. It was Kim's Gethsemane. She knew God was about to take her to Himself, and she didn't want to go. Her prayers mingled with ours that God would heal her and free her from this destiny. "Mrs. Mellecker, I'm not getting any better, and I'm so scared." I prayed a different prayer for Kim that night. "Lord, give her peace; don't let her be scared." Kim did receive that peace we prayed for. Like Jesus, she prayed to be spared this premature death. She wanted to live and have a home and family, and yet she was so faithful in accepting God's will over her own. She never pouted about it. If she had, she could not have been a successful witness, right to the moment when the Lord came for her.

Kim was a surrendered, faithful Christian, and as lightly as some of us take that title, Kim bore it with sparkle and courage. Her life was a witness to people she never even met. The Lord is using Kim's life, even now, as I share it with others.

Our family feels it was an honor to have known your

daughter. I pray that God will bless and sustain you who are left while Kim is in heaven—where I am sure Jesus has welcomed her with the words, "Well done, Kim, my good and faithful servant."

THE LEROY MELLECKER FAMILY

God, there was so much about this child of mine that I did not know! Leukemia allowed fear to cloud my understanding, anxiety to dull my perception, and tears to obscure my vision.

Three long years passed before my shell of grief began to crack and fall away.

The love I gave to Kim is one that needs to be given to many. It is a reversal procedure: from looking inward, to looking and producing outward. I've finally come to realize that it is not a matter of "getting myself together," but of "getting myself out," turning my energies toward meeting the needs of others.

Grief is now a part of my secret inner life. My laughter is real. My interest in others is real. My tears are real. I am no longer shackled by pretense. It takes determination and enthusiastic imagination to present an optimistic personality to the world. But, in giving, I am receiving. For the first time, I am beginning to look forward to the "good new days" with anticipation of fulfillment that the "good old days" could have never produced.

I have forgiven death for too soon taking from me my child, whom I needed so much. I have forgiven life for the supreme hurt. Death has become acceptable. But sorrow never leaves one at the same place she is found. What has emerged is a new me, reaching out for the riches of nonmaterialistic values, stronger, softer, and more understanding.

I look down and lovingly touch the gold and diamond #1 on a delicate chain around my neck, a Christmas gift from Jim and Jame. Closing my eyes, I hear Kim's voice once more, "Mom, good ol' mom. Next to God, you're number one."

With glistening eyes, I look up at the new calendar hanging on my pantry door, turned to January 1979. Through my tears, I smile.

Yesterday is not to be forgotten. It is to be cherished and remembered. But tomorrow? Tomorrow is to be created.

> Alas for him who never sees
> The stars shine through his cypress trees!
> Who, hopeless, lays his dead away,
> Nor looks to see the breaking day
> Across the mournful marbles play.
> Who hath not learned in hours of faith,
> The truth to flesh and sense unknown,
> That Life is ever Lord of Death,
> And Love can never lose its own!"
>   JOHN GREENLEAF WHITTIER

pull
5-30

1953 88